1000 EMQs for PLAB

BASED ON CURRENT EXAMS

Third Edition

SHERIF W HELMY

MBBCh, MRCP (UK), MRCGP

General practitioner with a special interest in cardiology
London

Foreword by
PROFESSOR SIR MAGDI YACOUB

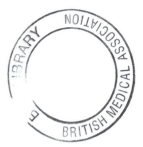

Radcliffe Publishing
London • New York

Radcliffe Publishing Ltd
33–41 Dallington Street
London
EC1V 0BB
United Kingdom

www.radcliffepublishing.com

British Library Cataloguing in Publication Data

A catalogue record for this book is available from the British Library.

ISBN-13: 978 184619 561 7

The paper used for the text pages of this book is FSC® certified. FSC (The Forest Stewardship Council®) is an international network to promote responsible management of the world's forests.

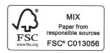

Typeset by Darkriver Design, Auckland, New Zealand
Printed and bound by TJI Digital, Padstow, Cornwall, UK

Contents

Foreword to the Third Edition

There is a continuing pressing need to enhance patient care globally through higher education. An essential part of achieving this for foreign graduates is the Professional and Linguistic Assessments Board (PLAB) test. Passing this test requires familiarity with its format.

In this book by Dr Sherif Helmy, a step-by-step approach to the test is presented in a lucid, easy-to-read format with comprehensive coverage of the subject. Dr Helmy has been kind enough to donate a major part of the proceeds of the book to the Chain of Hope charity, which is dedicated to establishing sustainable cardiac units in developing countries and is designed to save many lives.

Passing tests and obtaining qualifications is a prerequisite to helping different communities wherever they are.

Professor Sir Magdi Yacoub
September 2011

Preface to the Third Edition

This book aims to serve as a useful tool in preparing for the PLAB test and medical finals in the UK. It contains 1000 extended matching questions (EMQs) written in the same format as the actual test. I have made a few changes from the previous edition in view of subsequent changes in investigations and treatment. The most important addition to this edition is the inclusion of explanations for model answers, as requested in feedback on the previous edition. I have also replaced some old questions with modern queries, with up-to-date answers, to the best of my ability, bearing in mind the great pace of innovations in medicine.

The EMQs in this book have been carefully selected to cover all clinical specialities. Most of the EMQs are similar to those in the actual test. You will notice that certain topics are covered more extensively than others, in view of their clinical relevance.

It is of vital importance to concentrate on all the details given in the questions, e.g. age, occupation, past medical history and results of investigations. Such details can significantly influence the answers. I have tried to provide some direction in the phrasing of questions, as many questions can be deliberately vague and the answer can depend on a hidden clue. You will come across several questions where there could easily be more than one answer, e.g. choice of investigations. In such questions, choose the most relevant answer, e.g. the investigation that is most commonly used or that would confirm the diagnosis.

The best way in which to maximise the benefit obtained from this book is to read more about the topics here in a reference book, as this publication is not intended for use as reference. However, by covering all the topics in this book, you will hopefully avoid any surprises in the actual exam.

Finally, I wish all candidates sitting the PLAB test the best of luck on the day and a bright medical career in the UK.

Sherif W Helmy
September 2011

About the author

Sherif W Helmy passed the PLAB test in 1999, MRCP in 2002 and MRCGP in 2005. He trained in the West Midlands, Surrey and London. He is currently a GP in Hampstead and a GP with a special interest in cardiology in Westminster, working in association with St Mary's Hospital, London. He is also a GP appraiser for Camden and Westminster PCTs.

Acknowledgements

I am very grateful for the feedback, both positive and negative, on the previous edition. I have responded to requests for more emphasis on explanations rather than just the provision of answers. Obviously, in clinical practice reaching a diagnosis is a complex process where it is difficult to be absolutely certain, and that degree of uncertainty is reflected in the questions and answers provided in this book.

I am very grateful for the great support of my family during the prolonged preparation of this book. I am also grateful for the support of my colleagues in general practice, the Cardiology Department at St Mary's Hospital and Dr Emil Guirguis.

I wish to thank Gillian Nineham, Jamie Etherington and Radcliffe Publishing, and also Camille Lowe at Undercover project management for the great support that made it possible to publish this book. Finally, I wish to thank Professor Sir Magdi Yacoub for his kind foreword.

To Christine, David and Sofia

Themes

Theme: Breathlessness

Options

    A. Inhaled foreign body
    B. Anaemia
    C. Pulmonary oedema
    D. Bronchogenic carcinoma
    E. Extrinsic allergic alveolitis
    F. Pneumothorax
    G. Pulmonary embolism
    H. Pneumonia
    I. Bronchial asthma
    J. Pleural effusion
    K. Cryptogenic fibrosing alveolitis

Instructions

For each case, choose the single most appropriate diagnosis from the list of options above. Each option may be used once, more than once or not at all.

1. A 52-year-old woman on HRT presents with a swollen left calf, chest pain and shortness of breath.
2. A 78-year-old man has been short of breath for a few weeks. His chest radiography shows a right basal shadow rising towards the axilla.
3. A 54-year-old woman presents with a 9-month history of progressive breathlessness and cyanosis. Clinical examination reveals clubbing and bilateral inspiratory crackles.
4. A 27-year-old farmer presents with fever, malaise, cough and breathlessness, which he has had for a few days. His symptoms were worse in the evening. Clinical examination demonstrated coarse end-inspiratory crackles.
5. A 34-year-old tall, slim porter presents with sudden-onset chest pain and breathlessness. He had had similar episodes in the past.
6. A 76-year-old man presents with acute breathlessness, cough, frothy bloodstained sputum and palpitations. He is apyrexial. O/E: bilateral end-inspiratory crackles. ECG shows sinus tachycardia. Bilateral calf Doppler ultrasound scans reveals no abnormality.

Theme: Liver disease

Options

- A. Wilson's disease
- B. Primary sclerosing cholangitis
- C. Primary biliary cirrhosis
- D. Haemochromatosis
- E. Galactosaemia
- F. Gaucher's disease
- G. Dubin–Johnson syndrome
- H. Gilbert's syndrome
- I. Hepatocellular carcinoma
- J. Pancreatic carcinoma
- K. Chronic active hepatitis

Instructions

For each case, choose the single most appropriate diagnosis from the list of options above. Each option may be used once, more than once or not at all.

7 A 48-year-old man presents with a dull aching pain in the right hypochondrium, which he has had for 3 weeks. Other complaints include impotence, arthritis, lethargy and weight loss.

8 A 47-year-old alcoholic presents with weight loss, fever, ascites and pain in the right hypochondrium. Abdominal ultrasound shows a focal lesion in a cirrhotic liver. Serum AFP is grossly elevated.

9 A 41-year-old man with known ulcerative colitis presents with progressive abdominal pain and itching. On examination he was jaundiced.

10 A 35-year-old woman presents with jaundice and painless depigmented patches on her hands, neck and face. On examination multiple spider naevi were noted.

11 A 4-week-old baby was seen with vomiting, diarrhoea and failure to thrive. On examination there was hepatomegaly.

12 A 27-year-old nurse presents with jaundice a few weeks after starting oral contraception. She gave no history of exposure to halothane. Hepatitis serology was negative. Alanine aminotransferase (ALT) and aspartate aminotransferase (AST) were normal but urine showed bilirubinuria.

Theme: Causes of haematemesis

Options

A. Duodenal ulcer
B. Vascular malformation
C. Mallory–Weiss tear
D. Oesophageal varices
E. Gastric carcinoma
F. Crohn's disease
G. Oesophageal carcinoma
H. Haemophilia
I. Gastric ulcer
J. Oesophagitis
K. Meckel's diverticulum

Instructions

For each case, choose the single most appropriate diagnosis from the list of options above. Each option may be used once, more than once or not at all.

13 A 53-year-old unemployed alcoholic presents with haematemesis, a history of alcoholic liver disease and ascites.

14 A 77-year-old man with a history of dysphagia, mainly to solid food, and weight loss for 4 months.

15 A 59-year-old bank manager with a long history of indigestion presents with haematemesis, severe constant epigastric pain and weight loss.

16 A 34-year-old man presents with haematemesis, a history of back pain, arthritis, diarrhoea and weight loss.

17 A 37-year-old labourer presents to A&E with haematemesis after an episode of severe coughing. On examination he was very drunk and drowsy but there were no signs of chronic liver disease.

18 A 42-year-old secretary presents with haematemesis. She also complains of epigastric pain, which usually occurs at night. The pain is relieved by antacids and is worse when she is hungry.

Theme: Neurological disorders

Options

A. Subdural haematoma
B. Guillain–Barré syndrome
C. Frontal lobe abscess
D. Brainstem haemorrhage
E. Petit mal epilepsy
F. Multiple sclerosis
G. Idiopathic (benign) intracranial hypertension
H. Arnold–Chiari malformation
I. Meningitis
J. Normal pressure hydrocephalus
K. Motor neurone disease

Instructions

For each case, choose the single most appropriate diagnosis from the list of options above. Each option may be used once, more than once or not at all.

19 A 37-year-old engineer who was started on diuretics 2 months ago for hypertension attended a follow-up appointment with his GP and his blood pressure was 190/110 mmHg. His GP requested further investigations, but within 24 hours he was admitted to A&E with vomiting, acute vertigo and gross incoordination. On examination there was bilateral nystagmus.

20 A 78-year-old hypertensive woman is referred for fluctuating level of consciousness. On examination her blood pressure is 175/110 mmHg, fundus examination shows some hypertensive changes, her reflexes are bilaterally brisk and her plantars are upgoing.

21 A 26-year-old presents with a week's history of headache and diplopia. On examination she is obese and fundoscopy shows bilateral papilloedema.

22 A 28-year-old diplomat presents with sudden blurring of the left eye. A week earlier he had noted progressive clumsiness of the right hand. A few months earlier he had had an episode of left leg stiffness that resolved spontaneously.

23 A 19-year-old soldier is brought semiconscious to A&E. He has been complaining of severe headache and vomiting for a day. On examination there is widespread maculopapular rash all over his body.

24 A 36-year-old previously fit man developed a flu-like illness, which was followed 2 days later by burning pain in both legs. He later developed urinary retention and diplopia. On examination his straight-leg-raising test was positive bilaterally, ocular mobility was limited bilaterally but sensation was intact.

Theme: Mass in the right iliac fossa

Options

A. Appendicular mass
B. Tuberculosis
C. Crohn's disease
D. Ulcerative colitis
E. Caecal carcinoma
F. Lymphoma
G. Ectopic kidney
H. Tubo-ovarian mass
I. Ectopic pregnancy
J. Intussusception
K. Volvulus

Instructions

For each case, choose the single most appropriate diagnosis from the list of options above. Each option may be used once, more than once or not at all.

25 A 20-year-old Somali man presents with a 2-month history of weight loss, fever and mass in the right iliac fossa (Hb 10 g/dL, WCC 13 000/mm³, ESR 90 mm/h).

26 A 20-year-old Greek man presents with a 4-month history of weight loss, fever, night sweats and right-side abdominal pain. The pain usually follows alcohol intake. Clinical examination reveals a mass in the right iliac fossa.

27 A 70-year-old woman presents with nausea, increasing dyspepsia and a mass in the right iliac fossa (Hb 9.8 g/dL, MCV 65 fL).

28 A 25-year-old man is found to have a mobile mass in the right iliac fossa during a routine medical examination for insurance purposes.

29 A 25-year-old man presents with a 3-month history of central colicky abdominal pain associated with occasional vomiting and diarrhoea. A barium follow-through demonstrates the string sign of the terminal ileum, and clinical examination reveals a mass in the right iliac fossa.

Theme: Weight loss

Options

A. Thyrotoxicosis
B. Anorexia nervosa
C. Bulimia nervosa
D. Diabetes mellitus
E. Ascaris infestation
F. Bronchogenic carcinoma
G. Lymphoma
H. Coeliac disease
I. Ulcerative colitis
J. Pneumonia
K. Depression
L. Multiple myeloma

Instructions

For each case, choose the single most appropriate diagnosis from the list of options above. Each option may be used once, more than once or not at all.

30 A 19-year-old model presents with amenorrhoea for 3 months. Examination reveals that her BMI is 17. She denies having any problems related to her diet, though she feels that she is overweight. She specifically denies vomiting or diarrhoea.

31 A 45-year-old businessman presents with a 2-month history of intermittent fever and weight loss. He denies any pain or cough. Examination revealed generalised lymphadenopathy. Blood tests revealed an ESR of 110 mm/h with a normal full blood count, liver function, renal function and bone profile.

32 A 22-year-old nurse presents with a 6-month history of diarrhoea, bloating, fatigue and weight loss of 2 kg. She denies rectal bleeding but reports that her stools have been bulky and greasy.

33 A 60-year-old heavy smoker presents with a 3-month history of polydipsia, polyuria and weight loss. Fasting blood glucose level was 5.7 mmol/L. Corrected serum calcium level was 2.9 mmol/L.

Theme: Causes of pneumonia

Options

- A. *Staphylococcus aureus*
- B. *Cryptococcus*
- C. *Streptococcus pneumoniae*
- D. *Legionella pneumophila*
- E. *Mycobacterium avium-intracellulare*
- F. *Mycoplasma pneumoniae*
- G. *Pneumocystis jirovecii (carinii)*
- H. *Chlamydophila psittaci*
- I. *Escherichia coli*
- J. *Pseudomonas aeruginosa*
- K. *Mycobacterium tuberculosis*

Instructions

For each case, choose the single most appropriate causative organism from the list of options above. Each option may be used once, more than once or not at all.

34 A 37-year-old man presents with dyspnoea, cough, weight loss and night sweats. His chest radiograph shows diffuse bilateral infiltration.

35 A 48-year-old man presents with fever, rigors, headache and diarrhoea. He has recently been on holiday abroad. His chest X-ray shows consolidation.

36 A 24-year-old man presents with dry cough, skin manifestations, and bone and muscle aches. His chest radiograph shows widespread patchy shadows. Blood tests show evidence of haemolysis.

37 A 45-year-old farmer presents with flu-like illness, anorexia and dry cough. His chest radiograph shows patchy consolidation.

38 A 41-year-old drug abuser presents with fever, cough and breathlessness. This was preceded by viral influenza. Chest radiograph shows multiple abscesses.

39 A 14-year-old student with cystic fibrosis rapidly deteriorated and developed acute respiratory failure while in hospital.

Theme: Anaemia

Options

- A. Iron deficiency anaemia
- B. Spherocytosis
- C. Autoimmune haemolytic anaemia
- D. Aplastic anaemia
- E. Sideroblastic anaemia
- F. Pernicious anaemia
- G. Anaemia of chronic disease
- H. Thalassaemia major
- I. Glucose-6-phosphate dehydrogenase (G6PD) deficiency
- J. Folate deficiency anaemia
- K. Sickle cell anaemia

Instructions

For each case described below, choose the single most appropriate diagnosis from the list of options above. Each option may be used once, more than once or not at all.

40 A 49-year-old radiographer presents with pallor, recurrent infections and epistaxis.

41 A 46-year-old epileptic on phenytoin presents with marked pallor.

42 A 14-year-old girl presents with fatigue. Her father was diagnosed in his youth as having recurrent anaemia. On examination she is pale with a tinge of jaundice. The tip of her spleen is palpable.

43 A 78-year-old man presents with night fever, night sweats, easy fatiguability and pallor. On examination he has generalised lymphadenopathy and a large spleen.

44 A 12-year-old Greek boy with dysmorphic features was treated for 8 weeks with oral iron for anaemia without response. His blood film was dimorphic.

45 A 29-year-old man who is being treated for ulcerative colitis presents with pallor. His blood film shows reticulocytosis, fragmentation and Heinz bodies.

Theme: Nail lesions

Options

A. Psoriasis
B. *Pseudomonas* nail infection
C. Onychomycosis
D. Onychogryphosis
E. Infective endocarditis
F. Lichen planus
G. Koilonychia
H. Yellow nail syndrome
I. Leuconychia
J. Beau's lines
K. Nicotine staining of the nails
L. Pyogenic granuloma
M. Melanoma

Instructions

For each case, choose the single most appropriate diagnosis from the list of options above. Each option may be used once, more than once or not at all.

46 A 39-year-old woman presents with a 12-month history of thick fragile nails in both hands. She also noted dry skin affecting her elbows and knees, which she managed with skin emollients.

47 A 60-year-old man presents with a 2-month history of transverse ridges affecting all his nails. He was hospitalised for pneumonia 3 months ago.

48 A 35-year-old woman presents with a 6-month history of a longitudinal depression in several fingernails, while toenails were much less affected. There is no history of trauma. She admits to a history of intermittent itchy rash on both wrists. Examination reveals white oral mucosal lesions.

49 A 92-year-old man living alone presents to A&E with chest pain. Cardiac examination was unremarkable, but it was noted that his toenails were significantly thickened, elongated and curved.

50 A 40-year-old vegan who is currently being investigated for uterine fibroids presents with concave nails.

51 A 60-year-old man presents with a 4-month history of a black painful nail. He thought that he had injured his finger when it first started as a small lesion beneath the nail, but the lesion expanded in size, lifted the nail and started to become painful.

Theme: Ovarian tumours

Options

    A. Mucinous cystadenoma
    B. Corpus luteum cysts
    C. Endometrial cysts
    D. Teratoma
    E. Primary ovarian carcinoma
    F. Serous cystadenoma
    G. Retention cysts
    H. Arrhenoblastoma
    I. Ovarian fibroma
    J. Granulosa-theca cell tumour
    K. Polycystic ovaries

Instructions

For each description, select the single most appropriate diagnosis from the list of options above. Each option may be used once, more than once or not at all.

52 The most common virilising tumour of the ovary. It secretes androgens.

53 Large multi-cavity ovarian cyst, filled with thick fluid. It may reach a huge size occupying the whole peritoneal cavity.

54 Single-cavity ovarian cyst, filled with watery fluid. It is often bilateral and is potentially malignant.

55 Small, solid and hard, white benign tumour. It is usually unilateral and may be associated with ascites and pleural effusion.

56 It may contain sebaceous fluid, hair and teeth. It may be benign or malignant.

57 It causes excessive oestrogen production. It may occur at any age, causing precocious puberty in children, metrorrhagia in adults and postmenopausal bleeding in older women.

Theme: Causes of acute pancreatitis

Options
- A. Gallstones
- B. Hypertriglyceridaemia
- C. Mumps
- D. Alcohol
- E. Polyarteritis nodosa
- F. Hypothermia
- G. Cystic fibrosis
- H. Pancreatic carcinoma
- I. Iatrogenic
- J. Thiazide diuretics
- K. Hypercalcaemia

Instructions

For each case described below, choose the single most appropriate cause from the list of options above. Each option may be used once, more than once or not at all.

58 A 10-year-old girl with a history of recurrent chest infections and sinusitis presents with acute abdominal pain.

59 A 45-year-old obese woman with a history of recurrent pain in the right hypochondrium.

60 A 38-year-old driver presents with recurrent central abdominal pain, diarrhoea and bleeding per rectum. Three weeks earlier, he had had a flu-like illness with productive cough and myalgia. Chest examination shows bilateral inspiratory wheezes.

61 A 65-year-old man presents with progressive jaundice, anorexia and weight loss.

62 A 49-year-old woman presents with polyuria, haematuria, abdominal pain and bone aches. On examination her blood pressure is 170/100 mmHg.

63 A 12-year-old student presents with fever, anorexia, headache, malaise and trismus.

Theme: Cardiac lesions

Options

- A. Mitral stenosis
- B. Atrial septal defect
- C. Fallot's tetralogy
- D. Aortic stenosis
- E. Hypertrophic cardiomyopathy
- F. Mitral regurgitation
- G. Tricuspid stenosis
- H. Aortic regurgitation
- I. Tricuspid regurgitation
- J. Pulmonary stenosis
- K. Ventricular septal defect

Instructions

For each set of clinical findings, choose the single most appropriate diagnosis from the list of options above. Each option may be used once, more than once or not at all.

64 Slow rising carotid pulse, prominent left ventricular impulse, ejection click, ejection systolic murmur and fourth heart sound.

65 Bounding carotid pulse, laterally displaced apex, ejection systolic murmur, early diastolic murmur and third heart sound.

66 Jerky carotid pulse, dominant 'a' wave in jugular venous pulse, double apical impulse, ejection systolic murmur at the base and pansystolic murmur at the apex.

67 Elevated jugular venous pressure, early diastolic opening snap, mid-diastolic murmur and loud first heart sound.

68 Elevated jugular venous pressure, displaced apex, pansystolic murmur at the apex and third heart sound.

69 Loud pansystolic murmur at the left lower sternal area, mid-diastolic flow murmur at the apex and loud second heart sound.

Theme: Skin rash

Options
- A. Scabies
- B. Measles
- C. Cellulitis
- D. Rubella fever
- E. Roseola infantum
- F. Erythema infectiosum
- G. Varicella zoster virus
- H. Kawasaki disease
- I. Rocky Mountain spotted fever
- J. Scarlet fever
- K. Meningococcal meningitis

Instructions

For each case, choose the single most appropriate diagnosis from the list of options above. Each option may be used once, more than once or not at all.

70 A 4-year-old boy presents with a vesicular rash that appears in crops.

71 A 5-year-old girl presents with a rash that started as a marked erythema of the cheeks.

72 A 14-year-old girl presents with intensely pruritic rash with pustules. On examination the rash is generalised but is more in the folds between the fingers and toes.

73 A 6-year-old boy presents with mild fever and maculopapular rash. His mother reported that the rash started on the face then became generalised. On examination there is palpable cervical and occipital lymphadenopathy.

74 A 9-year-old boy presents with conjunctivitis and maculopapular rash. The rash started on the head and spread downwards.

75 An 18-month-old girl is admitted to A&E with a 6-hour history of fever and lethargy. On examination her temperature is 38.9°C, blood pressure is 70/40 mmHg, respiratory rate is 30 per minute and pulse is 120 bpm. Examination also reveals a full fontanelle and a petechial rash.

Theme: Rectal bleeding in children

Options

- A. Meckel's diverticulum
- B. Eosinophilic colitis
- C. Intussusception
- D. Haemolytic–uraemic syndrome
- E. Lymphonodular hyperplasia
- F. Juvenile polyps
- G. Ulcerative colitis
- H. Crohn's disease
- I. Haemorrhoids
- J. Hirschsprung's disease
- K. Anal fissure

Instructions

For each case, choose the single most appropriate diagnosis from the list of options above. Each option may be used once, more than once or not at all.

76 A 15-month-old boy is admitted to A&E shocked. There is no history of diarrhoea, but he has been passing large amounts of melanotic stool. On examination he is anaemic.

77 A 4-year-old girl presents with bloody diarrhoea and crampy abdominal pain. Blood tests show anaemia and thrombocytopenia.

78 A 5-week-old infant presents with scanty streaks of fresh blood mixed with normal-coloured stools.

79 A 7-year-old boy presents with streaks of fresh blood on the side of normal-coloured stools and drops of fresh blood in the toilet. There is no history of abdominal or rectal pain.

80 A 14-year-old boy presents with a 2-week history of abdominal pain and severe watery diarrhoea, with occasional bright blood mixed with stools. He complains of poor sleep as he has about 20 motions per day. Examination reveals mild diffuse abdominal tenderness and perianal skin tags.

81 A 12-year-old girl presents with a 4-week history of rectal bleeding and frequent loose motions. She reported lower abdominal cramping during defecation but denied fever, rash, weight loss, arthritis or vomiting. Investigations showed anaemia but normal ESR, albumin and liver enzymes.

Theme: Arthritis

Options

    A. Rheumatoid arthritis
    B. Psoriatic arthropathy
    C. Systemic lupus erythematosus
    D. Septic arthritis
    E. Seronegative arthritis
    F. Pyrophosphate arthropathy
    G. Haemarthrosis
    H. Osteoarthritis
    I. Gout
    J. Hyperparathyroidism
    K. Erythema nodosum

Instructions

For each case, choose the single most appropriate diagnosis from the list of options above. Each option may be used once, more than once or not at all.

82 A 77-year-old woman presents with pain and varus deformity of both knees. She also complains of pain in both hips and hands.

83 A 72-year-old woman presents with pain in both knees. Knee radiography shows a rim of calcification of the lateral meniscus.

84 A 30-year-old woman presents with pain and morning stiffness of the small joints of both hands.

85 A 30-year-old flight attendant presents with gritty eyes, dysuria and painful knees especially during standing. He has just returned from Thailand.

86 A 78-year-old man presents with pain and swelling of the left first metatarsophalangeal joint. He was started on thiazide diuretics 3 weeks earlier.

87 A 22-year-old previously fit soldier presents with a red, hot, tender and swollen knee. Leg muscles show marked spasm.

Theme: Genetics

Options

A. Schizophrenia
B. Coeliac disease
C. Vitamin D-resistant rickets
D. Cystic fibrosis
E. Peptic ulcer
F. Familial adenomatous polyposis
G. Turner's syndrome
H. Frontal baldness (androgenetic alopecia)
I. Rheumatoid arthritis
J. Duchenne muscular dystrophy
K. Hodgkin's lymphoma

Instructions

For each mode of inheritance, choose the single most appropriate disorder from the list of options above. Each option may be used once, more than once or not at all.

88 Autosomal dominant
89 Autosomal recessive
90 X-linked dominant
91 X-linked recessive
92 Sex-linked inheritance
93 Polygenic inheritance

Theme: Clinical features of cardiac arrhythmias

Options

A. Sinus tachycardia
B. Sinus bradycardia
C. Atrial fibrillation
D. Ventricular tachcardia
E. Ventricular fibrillation
F. First-degree heart block
G. Second-degree heart block (Mobitz type 1)
H. Second-degree heart block (Mobitz type 2)
I. Third-degree heart block
J. Haemorrhage
K. Ventricular ectopics
L. Atrial ectopics

Instructions

For each case, choose the single most appropriate diagnosis from the list of options above. Each option may be used once, more than once or not at all.

94 A 35-year-old motorcyclist is brought to A&E by ambulance following a road traffic accident. He has an impaired level of consciousness and his blood pressure is 85/45 mmHg, while his pulse is 125 bpm, regular rhythm.

95 A 68-year-old man is admitted to CCU following an inferior myocardial infarction. His pulse is 40 bpm, regular rhythm.

96 A 24-year-old athlete attends a routine medical insurance health assessment. His resting pulse is 48 bpm with a regular rhythm and his blood pressure is 106/70 mmHg.

97 A 69-year-old diabetic man is found to have an irregular pulse with a rate of 110 bpm during his diabetic review. He admits to occasional palpitations.

Theme: Lump in the groin

Options

    A. Inguinal hernia
    B. Femoral hernia
    C. Saphena varix
    D. Spigelian hernia
    E. Hydrocele
    F. Inguinal lymphadenopathy
    G. Haematocele
    H. Femoral artery aneurysm
    I. Pantaloon hernia

Instructions

For each case, choose the single most appropriate diagnosis from the list of options above. Each option may be used once, more than once or not at all.

98 A 40-year-old woman presents with a lump in the left groin. The lump is not reducible and lies below and lateral to the pubic tubercle.

99 A 40-year-old woman who underwent varicose vein surgery recently presents with a lump in the groin. The lump disappears on lying down and transmits cough impulse. It lies just below the groin crease and medial to the femoral pulse.

100 A 60-year-old man presents with a swelling in the groin and the scrotum. Clinical examination reveals a reducible scrotal swelling, and it is not possible to get above it.

101 A 10-year-old boy presents with a firm lump in the left inguinal region. O/E: there is an infected insect bite on the left thigh.

Theme: Causes of clubbing

Options

- A. Bronchial carcinoma
- B. Inflammatory bowel disease
- C. Bronchiectasis
- D. Liver cirrhosis
- E. Bacterial endocarditis
- F. Empyema
- G. Congenital cyanotic heart disease
- H. Cryptogenic fibrosing alveolitis
- I. Mesothelioma
- J. Lung abscess
- K. Familial clubbing

Instructions

For each case, choose the single most appropriate diagnosis from the list of options above. Each option may be used once, more than once or not at all.

102 A 39-year-old lawyer presents with rheumatoid arthritis and breathlessness. Her chest radiography shows basal shadows.

103 A retired labourer in a shipbuilding yard presents with worsening dyspnoea and pleuritic pain. His chest radiography shows pleural effusion, and his pulmonary function tests show a restrictive ventilatory defect.

104 A 67-year-old man presents with loss of weight, cough, numbness and tingling in both hands and feet, and muscle weakness.

105 A 58-year-old woman presents with left upper quadrant abdominal pain, which she has had for 3 weeks. A week before admission, she had developed night sweats, dizziness and confusion. On examination her temperature is 38.7°C, pulse is 120 bpm and blood pressure is 140/60 mmHg. Abdominal examination showed splenomegaly.

106 A 40-year-old man presents with a 4-week history of lower abdominal discomfort, severe diarrhoea with occasional blood and mucus mixed with the stools.

107 A 9-year-old boy was unable to participate in physical education because of progressive shortness of breath. His mother also noted mild bilateral ankle swelling.

Theme: Skin lesions

Options

- A. Chickenpox
- B. Bullous pemphigoid
- C. Pityriasis versicolor
- D. Pityriasis rosea
- E. Erythema nodosum
- F. Stevens–Johnson syndrome
- G. Pemphigus vulgaris
- H. Erythema marginatum
- I. Henoch–Schönlein purpura
- J. Erythema multiforme
- K. Measles

Instructions

For each skin lesion, choose the single most appropriate diagnosis from the list of options above. Each option may be used once, more than once or not at all.

108 Herald patch: solitary patch with peripheral scaling, most commonly found on the trunk.

109 Target lesions: concentric rings due to a cell-mediated cutaneous lymphocytotoxic response.

110 Thick-walled bullae. Immunofluorescence studies show linear staining of IgG along the basement membrane.

111 Thin-walled bullae. Immunoflourescence studies show intercellular staining of IgG within the epidermis.

112 Target lesions with extensive mucous membrane involvement.

113 Umbilicated vesicles, pustules and crusts. Rash distribution is centripetal.

114 Koplik's spots: on the mucosa of the cheeks opposite the molar teeth.

Theme: Operations in gynaecology and their indications

Options

- A. Anterior colporrhaphy
- B. Marsupialisation
- C. Wertheim's hysterectomy
- D. Dilatation and curettage
- E. Salpingectomy
- F. Vulvectomy
- G. Ventrosuspension
- H. Laparoscopy
- I. Manchester repair
- J. Abdominal tubal ligation
- K. Vaginal flap urethroplasty

Instructions

For each clinical presentation, choose the single most appropriate operation from the list of options above. Each option may be used once, more than once or not at all.

115 Abnormal uterine bleeding, missed abortion or incomplete abortion

116 Carcinoma of the vulva

117 Cystourethrocele

118 Descent of the uterus and laxity of the vaginal walls

119 Urethral stricture

120 Blocked Bartholin's duct

Theme: Urinary problems in women

Options

- A. True incontinence
- B. Urinary tract infection
- C. Overflow incontinence
- D. Urge incontinence
- E. Frequency of micturition
- F. Stress incontinence
- G. Urethral syndrome
- H. Gonococcal urethritis
- I. Urethral prolapse

Instructions

For each statement below, choose the single most appropriate condition from the list of options above. Each option may be used once, more than once or not at all.

121 May be triggered by sexual intercourse.

122 Occurs when there is a fistulous communication between the urinary and genital tracts.

123 Occurs when the bladder is full to its limit but is unable to empty.

124 Occurs when there is a sudden increase in intra-abdominal pressure.

125 Occurs when the desire to void is followed almost immediately by voiding.

126 Commonly occurs after catheterisation for urinary incontinence or retention.

Theme: Chest radiography findings in congenital heart diseases

Options

- A. Atrial septal defect
- B. Coarctation of the aorta
- C. L-transposition of the great arteries
- D. Fallot's tetralogy
- E. D-transposition of the great arteries
- F. Patent ductus arteriosus
- G. Total anomalous pulmonary venous return
- H. Ventricular septal defect
- I. Persistent truncus arteriosus
- J. Pulmonary stenosis
- K. Aortic stenosis

Instructions

For each radiographic finding, choose the single most appropriate diagnosis from the list of options above. Each option may be used once, more than once or not at all.

127 'Snowman' sign

128 Egg-shaped heart

129 Boot-shaped heart

130 Convex left heart border

131 'Figure 3' sign

132 Concave main pulmonary artery segment and right aortic arch

Theme: Paediatric neurological disorders

Options

- A. Platybasia
- B. Duchenne muscular dystrophy
- C. Brain abscess
- D. Syringomyelia
- E. Glioblastoma multiforme
- F. Agenesis of the corpus callosum
- G. Arnold–Chiari malformation
- H. Cerebral lymphoma
- I. Klippel–Feil syndrome
- J. Medulloblastoma
- K. Tuberous sclerosis

Instructions

For each case, choose the single most appropriate diagnosis from the list of options above. Each option may be used once, more than once or not at all.

133 A 7-month-old infant with infantile spasms and delayed milestones.

134 A 19-year-old student presents with loss of pin-prick and temperature sensation over her shoulders and upper arms. Magnetic resonance imaging (MRI) of the spine showed a fluid-filled cystic cavity in the cervico-thoracic cord.

135 A 3-week-old infant with meningomyelocele presents with progressive head enlargement since birth.

136 A 6-year-old boy presents with clumsiness, abnormal gait and repeated falls. On examination he had prominent calf muscles and lumbar lordosis. He waddled slightly while walking. Deep tendon reflexes were depressed at the ankles.

137 A previously healthy 5-year-old girl presents with a 3-week history of morning headaches and unsteady gait. CT showed a lesion in the cerebellar vermis.

138 A 9-year-old boy presents with learning difficulties. On examination he was found to have axillary freckles and multiple café au lait spots.

Theme: Causes of syncope

Options

A. Anxiety
B. Münchausen syndrome
C. Ménière's disease
D. Epilepsy
E. Orthostatic hypotension
F. Hypoglycaemia
G. Stokes–Adams attack
H. Vasovagal syncope
I. Transient ischaemic attack
J. Carotid sinus syncope
K. Micturition syncope

Instructions

For each case, choose the single most appropriate diagnosis from the list of options above. Each option may be used once, more than once or not at all.

139 A 76-year-old man fell to the floor while standing in a long queue. He regained consciousness within 2 minutes. He was not incontinent of urine or stools.

140 A 29-year-old secretary had a blackout while working on the computer. She was drowsy for 24 hours after the episode.

141 A 79-year-old woman fell to the floor as she tried to get up from bed. She had recently been started on an angiotensin-converting enzyme (ACE) inhibitor for hypertension.

142 A 55-year-old diabetic collapsed on a long flight. On examination there was pallor and tachycardia.

143 A 71-year-old woman presents with hemiparesis and diplopia which resolved within 24 hours.

144 A 63-year-old man presents following several episodes of loss of consciousness. He usually regained consciousness within a few seconds after falling on the floor. He reported that such episodes were usually preceded by palpitations.

Theme: Autoantibodies

Options

    A. Anti-microsomal antibody
    B. Cytoplasmic anti-neutrophil cytoplasmic antibody (c-ANCA)
    C. Anti-double-stranded DNA
    D. Anti-parietal cell antibody
    E. Anti-acetylcholine receptor antibody
    F. Anti-endomysial antibody IgA
    G. Anti-smooth muscle antibody
    H. Anti-streptolysin
    I. Anti-mitochondrial antibody
    J. Perinuclear anti-neutrophil cytoplasmic antibody
    K. Rheumatoid factor

Instructions

For each condition, choose the single most appropriate autoantibody from the list of options above. Each option may be used once, more than once or not at all.

145 Systemic lupus erythematosus (SLE)
146 Coeliac disease
147 Rheumatoid arthritis
148 Hashimoto's thyroiditis
149 Myasthenia gravis
150 Primary biliary cirrhosis
151 Wegener's granulomatosis

Theme: Visual field defects

Options

- A. Optic chiasmal lesion
- B. Frontal lobe lesion
- C. Parietal lobe lesion
- D. Unilateral occipital lobe lesion
- E. Optic nerve lesion
- F. Bilateral occipital lobe lesion
- G. Ciliary ganglion lesion
- H. Temporal lobe lesion
- I. Edinger–Westphal nucleus lesion
- J. Pretectal nucleus lesion

Instructions

For each visual field defect, choose the single most appropriate anatomical lesion from the list of options above. Each option may be used once, more than once or not at all.

152 Bitemporal hemianopia

153 Contralateral homonymous hemianopia

154 Anton's syndrome

155 Ipsilateral mononuclear field loss

156 Lower homonymous quadrantanopia

157 Upper homonymous quadrantanopia

Theme: Renal calculi

Options

A. Percutaneous nephrolithotomy (PCNL)
B. Extracorporeal shock wave lithotripsy (ESWL)
C. Alkaline diuresis
D. Nephrectomy
E. Percutaneous nephrostomy
F. Expectant management
G. Acid diuresis
H. Intravenous antibiotics
I. Peritoneal dialysis

Instructions

For each case below, choose the single most appropriate management from the list of options above. Each option may be used once, more than once or not at all.

158 A 30-year-old pregnant woman (26 weeks) presents with septicaemia and abdominal pain. Investigations reveal an obstructed right kidney due to a 2-cm calculus. She is commenced on intravenous antibiotics.

159 A 40-year-old man presents with left-side renal colic. Intravenous urography (IVU) shows a 1-cm calculus in the upper third of the ureter. There is no complete obstruction. His symptoms fail to resolve on conservative management.

160 A 20-year-old man presents with renal colic secondary to a 1-cm cystine calculus.

161 A 30-year-old man presents to A&E with right-side renal colic. IVU shows a 4-mm calculus in the distal part of the ureter with no complete obstruction.

162 A 40-year-old woman is found to have a staghorn calculus in a non-functioning kidney.

163 A 60-year-old man presents with frequent attacks of left-side renal colic due to a 2.5-cm calculus in the renal pelvis. He has a cardiac pacemaker and is known to have a 6-cm aortic aneurysm.

Theme: Malnutrition and malabsorption

Options

- A. Scurvy
- B. Beriberi
- C. Pellagra
- D. Riboflavin deficiency
- E. Vitamin A deficiency
- F. Rickets
- G. Vitamin K deficiency
- H. Iron deficiency
- I. Vitamin B_{12} deficiency
- J. Folate deficiency
- K. Iodine deficiency

Instructions

For each case, choose the single most appropriate diagnosis from the list of options above. Each option may be used once, more than once or not at all.

164 A 7-year-old boy presents with night blindness.

165 A 57-year-old alcoholic presents with peripheral oedema and ascites.

166 A 91-year-old woman presents with spontaneous bruising and anaemia.

167 A 38-year-old woman who is currently being investigated for uterine fibroids presents with brittle nails and angular stomatitis.

168 A 58-year-old man who had ileal resection for Crohn's disease.

169 A 47-year-old woman with primary biliary cirrhosis presents with bruising.

Theme: Adverse effects of medications

Options

A. Nifedipine
B. Carbimazole
C. Rifampicin
D. Ampicillin
E. Propranolol
F. Ramipril
G. Co-trimoxazole
H. Simvastatin
I. Thiazide diuretic
J. Isoniazid
K. Propylthiouracil

Instructions

For each case, choose the single most appropriate medication from the list of options above. Each option may be used once, more than once or not at all.

170 A 69-year-old alcoholic was diagnosed with tuberculosis. He was started on some medications, then a few months later developed numbness and tingling in both feet.

171 A 63-year-old diabetic was prescribed a medication for newly diagnosed hypertension. She did not tolerate the medication because of dry persistent cough.

172 A 14-year-old boy presents to his GP with fever, rash and sore throat. The GP diagnosed tonsillitis and started him on an antibiotic. He later developed a blotchy purpuric rash all over his body.

173 A 52-year-old, who had had a triple bypass, complained of myalgia a few weeks after starting a new medication. His liver function tests were abnormal.

174 A 68-year-old was started on a medication for hypertension. He presented later with a tender swollen right first metatarsal joint.

175 A 48-year-old woman with recently diagnosed thyrotoxicosis presents with fever and sore throat.

Theme: Pelvic pain

Options
- A. Ectopic pregnancy
- B. Ruptured ovarian cyst
- C. Pelvic inflammatory disease
- D. Appendicitis
- E. Endometriosis
- F. Inflammatory bowel disease
- G. Degenerating fibroid
- H. Septic abortion
- I. Diverticulitis
- J. Ovarian hyperstimulation syndrome

Instructions

For each case, choose the single most appropriate diagnosis from the list of options above. Each option may be used once, more than once or not at all.

176 A 23-year-old woman presents with pelvic pain, fever and vaginal discharge. On examination there is marked lower abdominal and adnexal tenderness. There is also cervical motion tenderness.

177 A 30-year-old woman presents with primary infertility, pelvic pain, dyspareunia and dysmenorrhoea. On examination there is beading and tenderness of the uterosacral ligaments and the uterus is fixed and retroverted.

178 A 19-year-old woman presents with severe colicky pain in the right iliac fossa and vomiting. Her periods are regular and pregnancy test is negative. On examination her temperature is 37.8°C and there is guarding rigidity.

179 A 27-year-old woman is admitted with vaginal bleeding and pelvic pain. She missed her last period and has had early morning sickness over the last week. On examination her blood pressure is 100/60 mmHg, pulse is 110 bpm and she is apyrexial.

180 A 35-year-old woman under treatment for infertility presents with pelvic pain, weight gain and abdominal distension. On examination there is shifting dullness.

181 A 25-year-old woman presents with severe pelvic pain, vaginal bleeding and fever. She has a positive pregnancy test.

Theme: Staging of malignant tumours

Options

A. Endometrial carcinoma: stage IIA
B. Vaginal carcinoma: stage II
C. Endometrial carcinoma: stage IIIA
D. Cervical carcinoma: stage IIA
E. Cervical carcinoma: stage IIIA
F. Endometrial carcinoma: stage IB
G. Ovarian carcinoma: stage IB
H. Cervical carcinoma: stage IIIB
I. Vaginal carcinoma: stage III
J. Vulvar carcinoma: stage II
K. Ovarian carcinoma: stage IIA

Instructions

For each statement below, choose the single most appropriate tumour stage from the list of options above. Each option may be used once, more than once or not at all.

182 The carcinoma involves the cervix and upper vagina but has not extended to the lateral pelvic walls or to the lower third of the vagina, and there is no parametrial involvement.

183 The carcinoma involves the endocervical glands as well as the body of the uterus.

184 The carcinoma involves the cervix, pelvic sidewall and hydronephrosis or non-functioning kidney.

185 The carcinoma involves both ovaries with metastases to the uterus and tubes, but negative peritoneal cytology.

186 The carcinoma invades the serosa of the body of the uterus with positive peritoneal cytology.

187 The carcinoma involves the vagina and extends to the pelvic sidewall.

Theme: Pulmonary diseases in children

Options

A. Pulmonary sequestration
B. Asthma
C. Tuberculosis
D. Bronchopulmonary dysplasia
E. Bronchogenic cyst
F. Cystic fibrosis
G. Pulmonary arteriovenous fistula
H. Laryngomalacia
I. Massive pulmonary embolism
J. Tracheo-oesophageal fistula
K. Pulmonary haemosiderosis

Instructions

For each case, choose the single most appropriate diagnosis from the list of options above. Each option may be used once, more than once or not at all.

188 A 4-year-old girl presents with a history of recurrent pneumonia and failure to gain weight. On examination wheezes and crepitations were heard and her fingers showed clubbing.

189 A 7-week-old infant presents with a 6-week history of noisy breathing. It is inspiratory in nature and increases when the baby is crying or during respiratory infections. It disappears completely when the baby is asleep.

190 A 5-year-old child presents with a history of chronic left lower lobe pneumonitis. On contrast bronchography the area involved fails to fill, outlined by bronchi that are filled.

191 A 4-year-old child presents with a history of dyspnoea, cyanosis, clubbing, haemoptysis and epistaxis. On examination there is generalised telangiectasia. Blood tests show polycythaemia.

192 A 1-month-old child presents with coughing, especially with feedings, and recurrent chest infections.

193 A 6-year-old boy presents to A&E with dyspnoea, wheezing and cough. On examination he is slightly cyanosed. His respiratory rate is 30 per minute, blood pressure is 100/60 mmHg and pulse is 110 bpm.

Theme: Investigating pulmonary diseases in children

Options

- A. Barium swallow
- B. Pulmonary angiography
- C. Chest radiography
- D. Contrast bronchography
- E. CT of the chest
- F. Fibre-optic bronchoscopy
- G. Chest ultrasonography
- H. ECG
- I. Carotid Doppler ultrasound
- J. Sweat test
- K. Echocardiography

Instructions

For each indication, choose the single most appropriate investigation from the list of options above. Each option may be used once, more than once or not at all.

194 To guide needle thoracentesis to sample a pleural effusion.

195 To assess an infant with excessive salivation, choking, coughing, vomiting, and cyanosis coincident with the onset of feeding.

196 To evaluate a child with chronic cough and wheezing.

197 To differentiate a mediastinal mass from a collapsed lung.

198 To rule out pulmonary arteriovenous fistula.

199 To rule out laryngomalacia.

Theme: Adverse effects of medications

Options

    A. Metformin
    B. Third-generation cephalosporin
    C. Lamotrigine
    D. Bleomycin
    E. Amiodarone
    F. Tolbutamide
    G. Vancomycin
    H. Lithium
    I. Phenytoin
    J. Doxorubicin
    K. Digoxin

Instructions

For each case, choose the single most appropriate medication from the list of options above. Each option may be used once, more than once or not at all.

200 A 67-year-old newly diagnosed diabetic was found lying on the floor in his house. On examination he was pale, hypothermic and bradycardic. His blood results were as follows: bicarbonate 13 mmol/L, urea 7.7 mmol/L, sodium 136 mmol/L and potassium 5.1 mmol/L.

201 A 35-year-old epileptic complains of impaired balance and blurring of vision. On examination there is nystagmus.

202 A 72-year-old man under treatment for squamous cell carcinoma of the lung becomes progressively short of breath. On examination there are bilateral basal lung crepitations. Chest radiography shows evidence of lung fibrosis.

203 A 76-year-old woman with paroxysmal supraventricular tachycardia presents with impaired vision, cold intolerance and constipation.

204 A 37-year-old man being treated for bipolar disorder presents with polyuria and coarse tremors.

205 A 91-year-old woman presents with severe urinary tract infection. One week after starting treatment, she developed profuse offensive diarrhoea.

Theme: Liver disease

Options

- A. Gilbert's syndrome
- B. Chronic active hepatitis
- C. Gaucher's disease
- D. Galactosaemia
- E. Primary biliary cirrhosis
- F. Alcoholic liver cirrhosis
- G. Wilson's disease
- H. Haemochromatosis
- I. Cholecystitis
- J. Hepatic adenoma
- K. Hepatic amoebiasis

Instructions

For each case, choose the single most appropriate diagnosis from the list of options above. Each option may be used once, more than once or not at all.

206 A 37-year-old woman presents with generalised pruritis for 6 months. On examination she was tanned and there were spider naevi on her chest. The liver was palpable one finger-breadth below the costal margin as well as the tip of the spleen.

207 A 30-year-old woman presents with anorexia, weight loss, lethargy and arthralgia for 3 weeks. On examination she was pale and jaundiced. The liver was palpable two finger-breadths below the costal margin as well as the tip of the spleen. Test results were: ALP 150 U/L, AST 875 U/L, bilirubin 39 μmol/L, albumin 21 g/L, globulin 52 g/L.

208 A 29-year-old woman presents with acute abdominal pain. Her bowels were regular with normal stools. She was taking oral contraceptive pills. On examination there were no features of chronic liver disease. Pulse 120 bpm, blood pressure 90/50 mmHg and temperature 37.2°C. Her abdomen was tender with guarding. The right hepatic lobe was palpable.

209 A 40-year-old man presents with worsening limb twitches and facial tics. He has been an inpatient in a psychiatric hospital for the last 5 years. His father had a similar history and died in a psychiatric hospital.

210 A 32-year-old man presents with haematemesis and shock. On examination there were multiple surgical scars over both knees, the right hip and the right hypochondrium. His liver was palpable four finger-breadths below the costal margin.

211 A fit 17-year-old man developed a flu-like illness followed 3 days later by abdominal pain, nausea, vomiting and jaundice. All his blood tests were normal apart from increased unconjugated bilirubin.

Theme: Management of endometriosis

Options

A. Danazol therapy
B. Oestrogen replacement therapy
C. Expectant management
D. Methotrexate
E. Conservative endometriosis surgery
F. GnRH agonists
G. Progestogens
H. Cyclic oral contraceptives
I. Non-steroidal anti-inflammatory drugs (NSAIDs)
J. Radical endometriosis surgery

Instructions

For each case, choose the single most appropriate management from the list of options above. Each option may be used once, more than once or not at all.

212 A 27-year-old journalist presents with an established diagnosis of mild endometriosis. She states that she wants to travel for 3 years before considering a pregnancy.

213 A 23-year-old woman presents with a 7-month history of infertility. Diagnostic laparoscopy shows evidence of mild endometriosis with scattered cul-de-sac implants. She has no other infertility factors.

214 A 33-year-old computer programmer presents with a 4-year history of infertility. A laparoscopic diagnosis of moderate endometriosis is made. Scattered endometrial implants in the pelvis, a 1-cm endometrioma on the right ovary and adhesions between the tube and ovary on each side are found.

215 A 37-year-old woman has just undergone radical endometriosis surgery.

216 A 36-year-old woman with a long history of endometriosis presents with menorrhagia and severe pelvic pain. She is not keen on any surgical intervention.

217 A 22-year-old single student is diagnosed with mild endometriosis and dysmenorrhoea.

Theme: Investigating amenorrhoea

Options

A. Measurement of serum prolactin levels
B. Laparoscopy
C. Measurement of TSH levels
D. Measurement of gonadotrophin levels
E. Karyotyping
F. Measurement of progesterone levels
G. Measurement of serum testosterone levels
H. Skull radiography
I. Hysteroscopy
J. Intravenous pyelography
K. Pelvic ultrasound scan
L. Measurement of β-HCG level

Instructions

For each case, choose the single most appropriate investigation from the list of options above. Each option may be used once, more than once or not at all.

218 A 22-year-old woman with previously normal menstrual cycles presents with irregular cycles and weight gain. Serum prolactin levels are elevated.

219 A 23-year-old nulligravida stopped her oral contraceptive pills to conceive. She had a menstrual flow after the last pack of contraceptive pills, then was amenorrhoeic for 7 months. She is otherwise fit and healthy.

220 A 25-year-old primipara returns 8 months after delivery complaining of amenorrhoea. Her pregnancy terminated with a Caesarean section because of abruptio placentae and foetal distress, with estimated blood loss of 1500 mL from a transient coagulation problem.

221 A 15-year-old student presents with primary amenorrhoea. On examination she is short, has low set ears and a webbed neck.

222 A 26-year-old woman presents with amenorrhoea for 7 weeks, vaginal spotting and mild right lower quadrant pain. Her periods have always been irregular. On examination the uterus is of normal size and the right lower quadrant is tender. Her β-HCG level the day before was 1100 mIU/mL.

Theme: Tumour markers

Options

    A. Calcitonin

    B. Human chorionic gonadotrophin (HCG)

    C. CA 15-3

    D. Thyroglobulin

    E. CA 125

    F. Carcinoembryonic antigen (CEA)

    G. CA 19-9

    H. Prostate-specific antigen (PSA)

    I. S-100

    J. α-fetoprotein (AFP)

Instructions

For each tumour, choose the single most appropriate tumour marker from the list of options above. Each option may be used once, more than once or not at all.

223 Carcinoma of the head of the pancreas

224 Ovarian carcinoma

225 Breast carcinoma

226 Prostatic carcinoma

227 Hepatocellular carcinoma

Theme: Thyrotoxicosis

Options

- A. Radioactive iodine
- B. Subtotal thyroidectomy
- C. Propranolol
- D. Carbimazole
- E. Potassium iodide
- F. Thyroxine
- G. Corticosteroids
- H. β-blockers
- I. Radiotherapy
- J. Total thyroidectomy
- K. Total thyroid lobectomy

Instructions

For each case, choose the single most appropriate management from the list of options above. Each option may be used once, more than once or not at all.

228 A 26-year-old pregnant woman is found to have thyrotoxicosis due to Graves' disease during the second trimester of the pregnancy. Her thyroid gland is very slightly enlarged.

229 A 15-year-old girl presents with thyrotoxicosis. A radioisotope scan shows an enlarged thyroid with uniform uptake throughout. She developed a keloid scar following an appendicectomy 2 years earlier.

230 A 30-year-old woman was diagnosed with Graves' disease. She remains thyrotoxic despite treatment with carbimazole for 1 year. In addition, she is currently troubled by her significantly enlarged thyroid.

231 A 60-year-old woman is found to have a large toxic nodular goitre.

232 A 50-year-old woman presents with thyroid enlargement. Thyroid function tests are normal. The needle biopsy confirms the diagnosis of Hashimoto's thyroiditis.

Theme: Chest radiography findings

Options

- A. Chickenpox pneumonia
- B. Mitral stenosis
- C. Consolidation
- D. Fallot's tetralogy
- E. Bronchiectasis
- F. Long-standing atrial septal defect
- G. Asbestosis
- H. Sarcoidosis
- I. Left ventricular failure
- J. *Pneumocystis jirovecii (carinii)* pneumonia
- K. Pulmonary embolus

Instructions

For each set of chest radiographic findings, choose the single most appropriate diagnosis from the list of options above. Each option may be used once, more than once or not at all.

233 Multiple calcified nodules mainly in the lower and mid zones. The nodules are less than 3 mm in diameter.

234 Multiple ring shadows at both lower lobes, giving a 'bunches of grapes' appearance with tramline shadowing.

235 Kerley B lines at each base and bilateral pleural effusion, together with hilar shadows.

236 Uniform well-defined shadow in the right upper lobe. Air bronchogram is also visible.

237 Double shadow at the right heart border and elevation of the left main bronchus.

238 Cardiomegaly, prominent right atrium, dilated pulmonary arteries and small aortic knuckle.

Theme: Anaemia

Options

- A. Pernicious anaemia
- B. Glucose-6-phosphate dehydrogenase (G6PD) deficiency
- C. Sickle cell anaemia
- D. Hereditary spherocytosis
- E. Thalassaemia major
- F. Anaemia of chronic disease
- G. Autoimmune haemolytic anaemia
- H. Macrocytic anaemia
- I. Paroxysmal nocturnal haemoglobinuria
- J. Iron deficiency anaemia
- K. Aplastic anaemia

Instructions

For each case described below, choose the single most appropriate diagnosis from the list of options above. Each option may be used once, more than once or not at all.

239 A 55-year-old woman with rheumatoid arthritis who is on non-steroidal anti-inflammatory drugs (NSAIDs) and steroids.

240 A 62-year-old male alcoholic with pallor, numbness and muscle weakness.

241 A 58-year-old woman with Addison's disease and peripheral neuropathy.

242 A 30-year-old man with abdominal pain and distension. Abdominal ultrasonography shows portal vein thrombosis.

243 A 57-year-old man with recently diagnosed non-Hodgkin's lymphoma presents with progressive pallor and dark urine.

244 A 27-year-old Italian waiter who becomes rapidly jaundiced after a course of ciprofloxacin.

Theme: Haematological diseases in children
Options
A. α-thalassaemia
B. Von Willebrand disease
C. Paroxysmal nocturnal haemoglobinuria
D. Iron deficiency anaemia
E. β-thalassaemia
F. Haemophilia A
G. Sickle cell anaemia
H. Glanzmann's thrombasthenia
I. Anaemia of chronic disease
J. Hereditary spherocytosis
K. Microangiopathic haemolytic anaemia

Instructions
For each of the following statements, choose the single most appropriate diagnosis from the list of options above. Each option may be used once, more than once or not at all.

245 Decreased haemoglobin, mean corpuscular volume (MCV), mean corpuscular haemoglobin (MCH) and mean corpuscular haemoglobin concentration (MCHC). Increased total iron binding capacity.

246 Reduced synthesis of α-globin chains leading to haemolysis.

247 Normal MCV. Decreased serum iron and total iron binding capacity. Increased serum ferritin.

248 It is due to a defect in spectrin and ankyrin.

249 Red blood cells unusually sensitive to the action of haemolytic complement.

250 Prolonged partial thromboplastin time (PTT) and bleeding time. Decreased ristocetin cofactor.

Theme: Paediatric oncology

Options

A. Wilms' tumour
B. Non-Hodgkin's lymphoma
C. Osteogenic sarcoma
D. Ewing's sarcoma
E. Medulloblastoma
F. Acute non-lymphocytic leukaemia
G. Neuroblastoma
H. Histiocytosis X
I. Acute bacterial lymphadenitis
J. Acute lymphoblastic leukaemia
K. Lymphoblastic lymphoma
L. Rhabdomyosarcoma

Instructions

For each case, choose the single most appropriate diagnosis from the list of options above. Each option may be used once, more than once or not at all.

251 A 3-year-old boy presents with a large left-side abdominal mass. Intravenous urography (IVU) shows a mass within the left kidney which encroaches on the collecting system. Chest radiography shows multiple pulmonary nodules.

252 A 10-year-old boy with diagnosed haemophilia presents with a 4-week history of enlarging left supraclavicular mass. The mass does not regress with factor VIII therapy.

253 A 12-year-old girl presents with a 3-day history of fever and a 3-cm warm, tender and fluctuant right anterior cervical lymph node.

254 An 18-month-old boy presents with periorbital echymoses and a large right loin mass. On examination he was anaemic and a large right-side mass distinct from the kidney is palpable. Bone marrow shows clumps of primitive cells. Bone scan shows increased activity in both orbits.

255 A 3-year-old girl presents with a 3-week history of morning headaches, vomiting and unsteady gait. CT shows a lesion in the cerebellar vermis.

256 A 14-year-old boy presents with a 2-week history of pain and swelling in the right thigh. Radiography of the right thigh shows a soft tissue mass with concentric layers of new bone formation. Blood tests reveal leucocytosis and elevated erythrocyte sedimentation rate (ESR).

Theme: ECG findings

Options

A. Right bundle branch block
B. Second-degree heart block (Mobitz type 1 – Wenckebach)
C. Hyperkalaemia
D. Pulmonary embolism
E. Sinus arrhythmia
F. Anterior myocardial infarction
G. Left bundle branch block
H. Wolff–Parkinson–White syndrome
I. Complete heart block
J. First-degree heart block
K. Second-degree heart block (Mobitz type 2)

Instructions

For each set of ECG findings, choose the single most appropriate diagnosis from the list of options above. Each option may be used once, more than once or not at all.

257 Progressive lengthening of PR interval with one non-conducted beat.

258 Constant PR interval but one P wave is not followed by a QRS complex.

259 One P wave per QRS complex, constant PR interval and progressive beat-to-beat change in RR interval.

260 Dominant R in V_1 and inverted T in the anterior chest leads.

261 Peaked P waves, right axis deviation, inverted T waves in leads V_1 to V_3 and tall R waves in V_1.

262 Dominant R waves in V_1, inverted T waves in leads V_1 to V_3 and deep S waves in V_6.

Theme: Psychiatric disorders
Options
- A. Depression
- B. Post-traumatic stress disorder
- C. Schizophrenia
- D. Chronic alcoholism
- E. Phobia
- F. Anxiety neurosis
- G. Mania
- H. Obsessive–compulsive disorder
- I. Depersonalisation
- J. Somatisation disorder (hysteria)
- K. Paranoid state

Instructions
For each case, choose the single most appropriate diagnosis from the list of options above. Each option may be used once, more than once or not at all.

263 A 23-year-old student presents with insomnia, headache, sweating, palpitations, chest pains and poor appetite.

264 A 35-year-old single woman presents with weight loss, poor appetite, decreased ability to concentrate and guilt feelings.

265 A 19-year-old female student presents with sudden blindness. Neurological examination reveals no abnormality.

266 A 20-year-old man presents with disinhibition, hyperactivity, increased appetite and grandiosity delusions.

267 A 30-year-old man presents with auditory hallucinations, social withdrawal and delusions of persecution.

268 A 21-year-old man presents with compulsions and rituals, which he resists.

Theme: Endocrine tumours

Options

A. Parathyroid adenoma
B. Multiple endocrine neoplasia (MEN) type 1
C. Multiple endocrine neoplasia (MEN) type 2
D. Carcinoid syndrome
E. Phaeochromocytoma
F. Medullary thyroid carcinoma
G. Parathyroid hyperplasia
H. Insulinoma
I. Follicular carcinoma of the thyroid
J. Prolactinoma
K. Pituitary adenoma secreting growth hormone

Instructions

For each case, choose the single most appropriate diagnosis from the list of options above. Each option may be used once, more than once or not at all.

269 A 40-year-old man presents with hypertension, palpitations and sweating; 24-hour urinary vanillylmandelic acid (VMA) is elevated. The lesion causing the symptoms is localised using an MIBG scan.

270 A 25-year-old woman presents with hypercalcaemia and bilateral nipple discharge. Serum parathyroid hormone and prolactin are elevated.

271 A 40-year-old man presents with recurrent episodes of flushing, colicky abdominal pain and asthma. Urinary 5-hydroxyindole acetic acid (5HIAA) is elevated.

272 A 45-year-old woman presents with hypercalcaemia and goitre. Investigations reveal elevated serum levels of parathyroid hormone and calcitonin. Past medical history includes a right adrenalectomy 3 years previously.

273 A 61-year-old woman presents with stiff joints, myopathy and constipation. Plain radiographs reveal a right renal calculus and evidence of osteitis fibrosa cystica.

Theme: Jaundice

Options

A. Primary biliary cirrhosis
B. Chronic active hepatitis
C. Carcinoma of the head of the pancreas
D. Primary sclerosing cholangitis
E. Primary hepatocellular carcinoma
F. Cholangiocarcinoma
G. Gilbert's syndrome
H. Dubin–Johnson syndrome
I. Stones in the common bile duct
J. Rotor's syndrome
K. Hepatitis A
L. Biloma

Instructions

For each case, choose the single most appropriate diagnosis from the list of options above. Each option may be used once, more than once or not at all.

274 A 12-year-old boy presents with jaundice after a recent episode of tonsillitis. Serum bilirubin rises further on fasting. Ultrasonography scan and liver biopsy reveal no abnormality.

275 A 27-year-old man presents with jaundice. He also describes a 6-month history of bloody diarrhoea. Haemoglobin is 10 g/dL, bilirubin is 75 μmol/L, and aspartate aminotransferase (AST), alanine aminotransferase (ALT), alkaline transferase (ALP) and gamma-glutamyl transferase (GGT) are all raised. Liver function tests improve with ursodeoxycholic acid.

276 A 45-year-old woman presents with painless jaundice 3 weeks after laparoscopic cholecystectomy. Bilirubin is 103 μmol/L, AST is 90 U/L and ALP is 760 U/L. She is apyrexial.

277 A 69-year-old woman presents with jaundice and backache. Clinical examination shows a mass in the right upper quadrant, acanthosis nigricans and superficial thrombophlebitis.

278 A 49-year-old woman with Sjögren's syndrome presents with jaundice and hepatosplenomegaly. Her urine is dark and serum contains antimitochondrial antibody (titre > 1 : 64); liver biopsy shows ductal destruction, proliferation and granuloma.

Theme: Causes of confusion

Options
- A. Dementia
- B. LSD abuse
- C. Hypothyroidism
- D. Post-ictal
- E. Alcohol withdrawal
- F. Subdural haemorrhage
- G. Meningitis
- H. Cerebral malignancy
- I. Hypoglycaemia
- J. Hyponatraemia
- K. Cerebrovascular accident

Instructions

For each case described below, choose the single most appropriate diagnosis from the list of options above. Each option may be used once, more than once or not at all.

279 A 70-year-old woman with tingling and numbness in her fingers, constipation and deafness.

280 A 22-year-old soldier with fever and rash.

281 A 69-year-old man with small cell (oat cell) carcinoma.

282 A 17-year-old student is brought by her friends to A&E at midnight with confusion. She is talking incoherently. Examination reveals dilated pupils and tachycardia.

283 A 20-year-old student who has been on insulin for 13 years.

284 A 79-year-old man is brought to A&E by his wife. He is unable to give any history, but his wife reports that she found him lying on the floor, rather confused. On examination he is incontinent of urine and stools and is bleeding from the mouth.

Theme: Drug overdose

Options

A. Lithium overdose
B. Aspirin overdose
C. Ethanol overdose
D. Benzodiazepine overdose
E. Tricyclic antidepressant overdose
F. LSD overdose
G. β-blocker overdose
H. Paracetamol overdose
I. Methanol overdose
J. Amphetamine overdose
K. Digoxin overdose

Instructions

For each case described below, choose the single most appropriate diagnosis from the list of options above. Each option may be used once, more than once or not at all.

285 A 19-year-old student was admitted to A&E with pyrexia and sweating. Her pulse was 120 bpm and blood pressure was 100/60 mmHg. She also complained of deafness and tinnitus.

286 A 34-year-old man was admitted to A&E unconscious. His temperature was 37.7°C, pulse was 130 bpm and blood pressure was 90/65 mmHg. Neurological examination showed bilateral extensor plantars. His pupils were dilated. ECG showed sinus tachycardia and occasional ventricular ectopics.

287 A 69-year-old man presents with drowsiness and confusion. His pulse was 48 bpm and his blood pressure was 98/68 mmHg. ECG showed first-degree heart block and widening of the QRS complex.

288 A 77-year-old woman presents with nausea, vomiting and diarrhoea. She also complained of blurring of vision and flashes of light. On examination she was slightly confused and her pulse was slow and irregular.

289 A 37-year-old woman with long-standing psychiatric illness was admitted with polyuria, diarrhoea, vomiting and coarse tremor involving both hands.

290 A 24-year-old waitress developed jaundice, right hypochondrial pain and tenderness, hypoglycaemia and oliguria 2 days after an overdose.

Theme: Haemoptysis

Options

    A. Pulmonary infarction
    B. Tuberculosis
    C. Mitral stenosis
    D. Foreign body inhalation
    E. Haemorrhagic telangiectasia
    F. Bronchogenic carcinoma
    G. Pneumonia
    H. Bronchiectasis
    I. Systemic lupus erythematosus (SLE)
    J. Wegener's granulomatosis
    K. Polyarteritis nodosa

Instructions

For each case, choose the single most appropriate diagnosis from the list of options above. Each option may be used once, more than once or not at all.

291 A 55-year-old smoker with a long history of recurrent chest infection presents with haemoptysis and greenish sputum. On examination he has clubbing and coarse crepitations over the bases of both lungs.

292 A 69-year-old woman who had a total hip replacement 1 week ago presents with severe chest pain, shortness of breath and haemoptysis.

293 A 52-year-old diabetic presents with fever, pleuritic pain and rusty-coloured sputum.

294 A 45-year-old bank manager presents with cough, pleuritic chest pain and haemoptysis. This was preceded by rhinitis, recurrent epistaxis and haematuria. Chest radiography shows multiple nodular masses.

295 A 69-year-old smoker presents with cough, haemoptysis and weight loss. On examination there is clubbing and gynaecomastia.

296 A 72-year-old Asian immigrant presents with cough, haemoptysis, night fever and sweating.

Theme: Human leucocyte antigens

Options

- A. Coeliac disease
- B. Acute pancreatitis
- C. Peptic ulcer
- D. Primary Sjögren's syndrome
- E. De Quervain's thyroiditis
- F. Primary biliary cirrhosis
- G. Insulin-dependent diabetes mellitus
- H. Motor neurone disease
- I. Myasthenia gravis
- J. Hydrocephalus
- K. Ankylosing spondylitis

Instructions

For each human leucocyte antigen shown below, choose the single most appropriate association from the list of options above. Each option may be used once, more than once or not at all.

297 *HLA*-B27
298 *HLA*-DR3
299 *HLA*-DR7
300 *HLA*-DR4
301 *HLA*-A3
302 *HLA*-DQ8

Theme: Therapeutics

Options

A. Oestrogens and progestins
B. Androgens
C. Prostaglandin inhibition
D. Hydrocortisone
E. Methotrexate
F. Progestational agents
G. Danazol
H. Clomiphene citrate
I. Diuretics
J. Tetracyclin
K. β-blockers

Instructions

For each diagnosis, choose the single most appropriate medication from the list of options above. Each option may be used once, more than once or not at all.

303 Congenital adrenal hyperplasia
304 Dysmenorrhoea
305 Dysfunctional uterine bleeding
306 Isosexual precocious puberty
307 Anovulation
308 Choriocarcinoma

Theme: Amenorrhoea

Options

A. Torsion of an ovarian cyst
B. Hydatidiform (vesicular) mole
C. Threatened miscarriage
D. Physiological amenorrhoea
E. Ectopic pregnancy
F. Androgen excess amenorrhoea
G. Bleeding corpus luteum
H. Hypogonadotrophic amenorrhoea
I. Eugonadotrophic amenorrhoea
J. Hypergonadotrophic amenorrhoea

Instructions

For each case, choose the single most appropriate diagnosis from the list of options above. Each option may be used once, more than once or not at all.

309 A 23-year-old woman whose last menses were 7 weeks ago presents with acute right lower quadrant pain. Serum β-HCG levels are elevated. Pelvic ultrasonography reveals no sac in the uterus and a 3 × 3 cm right adnexal mass.

310 A 28-year-old woman who is 18 weeks pregnant presents with painless vaginal bleeding. She has been complaining of hyperemesis gravidarum for several weeks. Serum β-HCG levels are low for dates. Pelvic ultrasonography reveals an intrauterine sac without foetal parts.

311 A 27-year-old whose last period was 8 weeks ago presents with heavy vaginal bleeding and left lower quadrant pain. Serum β-hCG is slightly elevated. Vaginal examination shows a closed cervical os.

312 A 14-year-old adolescent with normal sexual development complains of amenorrhoea for 5 months. Her first menses were 10 months ago, since which she has had three menses.

313 A 26-year-old nulligravida had a normal menstrual history until 9 months ago, when she began intensive long-distance running. She has not had a menstrual flow since her first marathon 5 months ago.

314 A 19-year-old woman with well-developed secondary sexual characteristics presents with amenorrhoea. She has a vaginal pouch, and karyotyping shows XX chromosomes.

Theme: Chest pain

Options

- A. Dissecting aortic aneurysm
- B. Dressler's syndrome
- C. Boerhaave's syndrome
- D. Ventricular aneurysm
- E. Pulmonary embolism
- F. Kawasaki disease
- G. Hypertrophic cardiomyopathy
- H. Pneumothorax
- I. Right ventricular infarction
- J. Cardiac neurosis
- K. Reflux oesophagitis

Instructions

For each case, choose the single most appropriate diagnosis from the list of options above. Each option may be used once, more than once or not at all.

315 A 56-year-old dentist had a successful operation for a fracture of the right neck of the femur. Six days later he complained of dyspnoea at rest and chest pain. ECG showed sinus tachycardia and right axis deviation.

316 A 60-year-old porter collapsed while bending to carry a bag. On admission to A&E, he regained consciousness but started to vomit and complained of severe stabbing chest pain. Chest radiography showed a widened mediastinum.

317 A 70-year-old man is admitted with severe epigastric pain and sweating. Over the last few weeks he has suffered from chest pain and shortness of breath on moderate exercise. On examination his jugular venous pressure (JVP) is 8 cm above the sternal angle, pulse is 65 bpm and blood pressure is 115/65 mmHg, and there is bilateral ankle oedema.

318 A 48-year-old alcoholic is admitted to A&E with severe retrosternal pain and shortness of breath. The pain is constant and radiates to the neck and interscapular region. On examination his pulse is 120 bpm, blood pressure is 90/60 mmHg and the left lung base is dull on percussion.

319 A 24-year-old engineer presents with worsening shortness of breath and chest tightness. His father had collapsed and died suddenly when he was 33. On examination the cardiac apex is double and both fourth heart sound and late systolic murmur are audible at the apex.

320 A 5-year-old boy presents with a history of high fever for a week and chest pain for a few hours. On examination his temperature was 38.8°C, pulse 110 bpm and blood pressure 100/60 mmHg; there was normal apex, cervical lymphadenopathy, erythematous buccal cavity and polymorphous rash.

Theme: Cerebrovascular disease

Options
- A. Transient ischaemic attack involving the carotid system
- B. Sagittal sinus thrombosis
- C. Extradural haemorrhage
- D. Lateral medullary syndrome
- E. Subarachnoid haemorrhage
- F. Subdural haemorrhage
- G. Cerebellar haemorrhage
- H. Lacunar infarction
- I. Hypertensive encephalopathy
- J. Pseudobulbar palsy
- K. Vertebrobasilar insufficiency

Instructions

For each case, choose the single most appropriate diagnosis from the list of options above. Each option may be used once, more than once or not at all.

321 A 73-year-old man recently diagnosed with atrial fibrillation presents with hemianopia, hemisensory loss, hemiparesis and aphasia of 16 hours' duration.

322 A 79-year-old man with a long history of diabetes and hypertension presents with vertigo that was triggered by suddenly looking upwards. Turning the head to the left reproduces vertigo.

323 A 60-year-old hypertensive and diabetic is admitted with acute dizziness, vomiting and difficulty in moving his right arm and leg. On examination there is Horner's syndrome on the right side.

324 A 58-year-old man presents to A&E with a severe headache and drowsiness which started suddenly while he was working on the computer. He had vomited once. On examination he was apyrexial, his pulse was 100 bpm and blood pressure was 160/100 mmHg.

325 A 72-year-old man was referred by his GP for recurrent headaches and fluctuating level of consciousness. There was no history of direct head trauma.

Theme: Lower limb ischaemia

Options
  A. Femoro-popliteal bypass
  B. Percutaneous balloon angioplasty
  C. Femoro-distal bypass
  D. Intra-arterial tissue plasminogen activator infusion
  E. Below-knee amputation
  F. Fasciotomy
  G. Lumbar sympathectomy
  H. Aorto-femoral bypass
  I. Axillo-femoral bypass
  J. Femoro-femoral crossover graft

Instructions

For each case, choose the single most appropriate procedure from the list of options above. Each option may be used once, more than once or not at all.

326 A 65-year-old man presents with intermittent claudication of the left calf. The claudication distance is 100 m. Angiography demonstrates a 1.5-cm stenosis of the left superficial femoral artery.

327 A 73-year-old diabetic woman presents with critical ischaemia of the right leg. Angiography reveals extensive disease of the superficial femoral, popliteal and tibial arteries. Pulse-generated run-off assessment indicates a good run-off in the posterior tibial artery.

328 A 72-year-old man presents with a 4-hour history of acute ischaemia of the left leg. Clinical examination reveals signs of acute ischaemia with no evidence of gangrene. There is no neurological deficit. An urgent arteriogram reveals a complete occlusion of the distal superficial femoral artery most likely caused by thrombosis.

329 A 57-year-old smoker presents with intermittent claudication of the right calf. The claudication distance is 70 m. Angiography reveals a 12-cm stenosis in the proximal superficial femoral artery.

330 A 21-year-old motorcyclist presents with multiple injuries following a road traffic accident. Clinical examination reveals a critically isch-aemic right lower leg. The right dorsalis pulse is feeble. The right calf is tense and swollen. The intracompartmental pressure is 55 mmHg. Angiography shows no discontinuity of the arterial tree.

Theme: Thyroid cancer

Options

A. Total thyroid lobectomy
B. Ablative dose of radioactive iodine
C. External beam radiation
D. Chemotherapy
E. Reassure and repeat fine needle aspiration cytology in 12 months
F. Thyroxine
G. Dexamethasone
H. Carbimazole
I. Subtotal thyroidectomy
J. Total thyroidectomy followed by radioactive iodine
K. Total thyroidectomy and complete central neck dissection

Instructions

For each case, choose the single most appropriate management from the list of options above. Each option may be used once, more than once or not at all.

331 A 40-year-old woman presents with symptoms of thyrotoxicosis. A thyroid ultrasound scan showed a solitary nodule in the right thyroid lobe. Fine needle aspiration cytology (FNAC) suggests follicular adenoma.

332 A 42-year-old woman presents with a 4-cm solid mass in the left thyroid lobe. FNAC reveals papillary carcinoma.

333 A 15-year-old boy presents with a 1-cm solitary thyroid nodule and diarrhoea. FNAC is reported as malignant. Serum calcitonin is raised.

334 A 30-year-old woman presents with a 2-cm thyroid nodule. FNAC suggests a colloid nodule.

335 A 50-year-old woman presents with a thyroid goitre. A core biopsy reveals evidence of lymphoma.

Theme: Inborn errors of metabolism

Options

A. McArdle's disease
B. Gaucher's disease
C. Fanconi's syndrome
D. Homocystinuria
E. Phenylketonuria
F. Galactosaemia
G. Hartnup disease
H. Cystinosis
I. Niemann–Pick disease
J. Cystinuria
K. Fabry's disease

Instructions

For each statement, choose the single most appropriate diagnosis from the list of options above. Each option may be used once, more than once or not at all.

336 Mental retardation and epilepsy. Urine analysis shows phenyl pyruvate.

337 Hepatosplenomegaly, pigmentation of exposed parts and anaemia.

338 Muscle cramps and myoglobinuria after exercise.

339 Hepatosplenomegaly, renal tubular defects, cataract and mental retardation.

340 Mental retardation, downwards subluxation of the lens, recurrent thrombosis.

341 Recurrent urinary stones.

Theme: Neurological disorders

Options

- A. Multiple sclerosis
- B. Lateral medullary syndrome
- C. Sagittal sinus thrombosis
- D. Guillain–Barré syndrome
- E. Motor neurone disease
- F. Arnold–Chiari malformation
- G. Normal pressure hydrocephalus
- H. Myasthenia gravis
- I. Herpes simplex encephalitis
- J. Peripheral neuritis
- K. Benign intracranial hypertension

Instructions

For each case, choose the single most appropriate diagnosis from the list of options above. Each option may be used once, more than once or not at all.

342 A 35-year-old clerk presents with diplopia and fatigue. Her symptoms are worse towards the evening.

343 A 33-year-old carpenter presents with unsteadiness of gait, incoordination of both arms and oscillopsia on down gaze. Clinical examination demonstrates a low hairline, positive Romberg's test and bilateral extensor plantars.

344 A 40-year-old woman presents with increasing weakness and stiffness of her legs. Three years ago she had had a similar episode, which lasted a few days and resolved on its own. A year later, she developed diplopia for 2 weeks.

345 A 70-year-old man presents with urinary incontinence and poor muscle coordination. On examination he is slightly confused, but apyrexial and there is no papilloedema. Two years ago he had meningitis which was successfully treated by antibiotics.

346 A previously fit 60-year-old lawyer is admitted to A&E with a 3-day history of progressively bizarre and aggressive behaviour. On examination she is confused and pyrexial. EEG shows abnormal complexes over the temporal lobe.

347 A 58-year-old man presents with progressive clumsiness and difficulty in performing fine tasks with both hands. On examination there is slight wasting of the intrinsic muscles of both hands, but more on the left. Reflexes and coordination are normal and there is no sensory deficit.

Theme: Renal impairment

Options

    A. Medullary sponge kidney
    B. Renal tubular acidosis
    C. Renal vein thrombosis
    D. Acute interstitial nephritis
    E. Bartter's syndrome
    F. Idiopathic hypercalciuria
    G. Diabetic nephropathy
    H. Cystinuria
    I. Renal artery stenosis
    J. Lupus nephritis
    K. Minimal change glomerulonephritis

Instructions

For each case, choose the single most appropriate diagnosis from the list of options above. Each option may be used once, more than once or not at all.

348 A 19-year-old mechanic was started on flucloxacillin for an infected wound. Blood tests done 3 days later showed evidence of renal failure. Urine was positive for blood and protein. Abdominal ultrasonography showed normal kidneys with no evidence of obstruction.

349 A 35-year-old woman presents with a blood pressure of 190/110 mmHg and impaired renal function. Urine microscopy showed scanty red cells and granular casts. Renal biopsy showed linear IgG on glomerular basement membrane.

350 A 40-year-old man presents with renal colic. He had had several similar episodes in the past which were sometimes associated with passing small stones. Abdominal radiography showed calcified opacities in both kidneys. All blood and urinary tests were normal.

351 A 7-year-old girl presents with renal colic. She was previously fit and had no family history of renal problems. Blood tests were all normal but urinary calcium was elevated.

352 A previously fit 17-year-old porter presents with renal colic. On examination his left flank was tender. Blood tests were normal. Urine microscopy showed hexagonal crystals. Intravenous pyelography (IVP) showed faintly opaque staghorn calculus in the left renal pelvis.

353 A 66-year-old diabetic woman was investigated for hyperkalaemia. She was on indomethacin and glibenclamide. Blood tests showed evidence of renal impairment, hyperkalaemia and hyperchloraemia.

Theme: Radiological investigations

Options

A. Radioisotope bone scan
B. MRI
C. Ultrasound scan
D. Duplex (Doppler) scan
E. CT scan
F. Angiogram
G. Lumbar puncture
H. Spiral (helical) CT scan

Instructions

For each statment, choose the single most appropriate investigation from the list of options above. Each option may be used once, more than once or not at all.

354 Is useful to assess renal size, identify parenchymal pattern and detect renal stones.

355 Is more sensitive for early space-occupying lesions, especially in the posterior cranial fossa.

356 Is contraindicated in a patient who is suspected to have a space-occupying lesion of the brain.

357 Is of great value in patients with possible pulmonary embolism and co-existing cardiorespiratory disease.

358 Is useful in demonstrating the cause of recurrent TIAs.

359 Is efficient in detecting osteolytic bony metastases.

Theme: Vaginal bleeding

Options

    A. Retention of a succenturiate lobe
    B. Placenta praevia
    C. Uterine rupture
    D. Cervical carcinoma
    E. Ruptured vasa praevia
    F. Cervical laceration
    G. Thrombocytopenia
    H. Implantation in the lower uterine segment
    I. Endometrial carcinoma
    J. Atonic uterus
    K. Placenta accreta

Instructions

For each case, choose the single most appropriate diagnosis from the list of options above. Each option may be used once, more than once or not at all.

360 Following a spontaneous vaginal delivery, a 22-year-old woman continues to bleed in spite of the use of oxytocin. The uterus appears to contract well but then relaxes with increased bleeding.

361 A 28-year-old woman has just delivered her second baby in 2 years after an oxytocin-induced labour. She is bleeding heavily despite the use of oxytocics. The uterus is well contracted and there is no evidence of vaginal or cervical tears. The baby weighs 4.5 kg.

362 A 32-year-old woman is still bleeding heavily 6 hours after having delivered twins vaginally.

363 A 40-year-old woman presents with a 3-month history of dyspareunia and post-coital bleeding. She has been a smoker for 20 years. She had had four normal deliveries and a miscarriage in the past. Her last smear was 3 years ago and showed mild dyskaryosis.

364 A 32-year-old woman presents in active labour with excessive vaginal bleeding. She has had a previous Caesarean section. The foetal heart rate is 65 bpm.

365 A 28-year-old woman who is 36 weeks pregnant presents with vaginal bleeding, contractions and a tender abdomen.

366 A 31-year-old woman has delivered with a complete placenta praevia by Caesarean section. Two hours later, she is noted to have significant post-partum haemorrhage.

Theme: Management of vaginal bleeding

Options

- A. Endometrial biopsy
- B. Combined oral contraceptive pill
- C. Myomectomy
- D. Dilatation and curettage
- E. Progesterone-only contraceptive pill
- F. Topical oestrogen
- G. Tranexamic acid
- H. Hysterectomy
- I. Oral iron therapy
- J. Hormone replacement therapy
- K. Laparoscopy

Instructions

For each case, choose the single most appropriate management from the list of options above. Each option may be used once, more than once or not at all.

367 A 46-year-old woman presents with a 1-year history of menometror-rhagia. On examination she is slightly obese, her uterus is of normal size and her blood pressure is 145/100 mmHg.

368 A 37-year-old woman presents with a 3-month history of menometror-rhagia. She has been on oral contraceptive pills.

369 A 22-year-old nulligravida presents with bleeding which has continued for 3 weeks, the last 4 days of which were heavy bleeding with clots. Her last menstrual period was 3 months before this bleeding episode. Her haemoglobin is 10.7 g/dL. Pregnancy test is negative.

370 A 32-year-old woman presents with menorrhagia. Her cycles are regular. On examination she is of average build, her uterus is of normal size and her blood pressure is 135/85 mmHg.

371 A 29-year-old primipara presents with a uterine mass and menorrhagia. On examination the uterus is a size appropriate to a 15-week gestation and a posterior fundal mass is found.

372 A 52-year-old woman with a known myomatous uterus presents with menometrorrhagia. She reports that her menses occur every 6 weeks and that she had had 5–8 days of intermenstrual spotting over the past four cycles.

Theme: Vascular disease

Options

A. Aorto-femoral bypass
B. Percutaneous transluminal angioplasty
C. Axillo-femoral bypass
D. Femoro-femoral crossover graft
E. Lumbar sympathectomy
F. Ileo-femoral bypass
G. Femoro-popliteal bypass
H. Femoro-tibial bypass
I. Fasciotomy
J. Below-knee amputation

Instructions

For each case, choose the single most appropriate operation from the list of options above. Each option may be used once, more than once or not at all.

373 A 70-year-old man presents with thigh claudication. Angiography demonstrates atherosclerotic narrowing of the distal aorta and proximal common iliac arteries.

374 An 83-year-old woman (a smoker) presents with left thigh and buttock claudication. Angiography reveals a smooth narrowing (1.5 cm in length) in the left common iliac artery.

375 A 75-year-old man presents with severe right calf claudication. Angiography shows narrowing (10 cm in length) of the right distal superficial femoral and popliteal arteries. The right posterior tibial artery has a reasonable run-off.

376 A 78-year-old man with severe emphysema presents with severe claudication of the left thigh and calf. Angiography reveals severe atherosclerosis affecting the left common and external iliac arteries. His past medical history includes previous anterior excision of the rectum and post-operative radiotherapy.

Theme: Skeletal pain

Options

A. Osteosarcoma
B. Ewing's sarcoma
C. Tuberculosis
D. Metastases
E. Multiple myeloma
F. Primary hyperparathyroidism
G. Osteoporosis
H. Osteomyelitis
I. Osteoarthritis
J. Septic arthritis

Instructions

For each case, choose the single most appropriate diagnosis from the list of options above. Each option may be used once, more than once or not at all.

377 A 70-year-old man presents with backache. Plain radiographs show multiple sclerotic areas in the lumbosacral spine.

378 A 50-year-old woman presents with backache and anaemia. Skeletal survey shows multiple lytic lesions in the skull and spine. Urine contains Bence Jones proteins.

379 A 15-year-old boy presents with a painful swelling around the left knee. A plain radiograph shows a lytic lesion with sunburst appearance.

380 A 60-year-old woman presents with backache. Plain radiographs reveal osteoporosis, bony cysts and subperiosteal bone resorption.

381 A 70-year-old man with a history of Paget's disease of bone presents with a painful swelling of the femur.

Theme: Breathlessness

Options

- A. Extrinsic allergic alveolitis
- B. Cystic fibrosis
- C. Cryptogenic fibrosing alveolitis
- D. Histoplasmosis
- E. Churg–Strauss syndrome
- F. Pneumothorax
- G. Allergic bronchopulmonary aspergillosis
- H. *Pneumocystis jirovecii* (*carinii*) pneumonia
- I. Goodpasture's syndrome
- J. Acute myocardial infarction
- K. Pulmonary embolism

Instructions

For each case, choose the single most appropriate diagnosis from the list of options above. Each option may be used once, more than once or not at all.

382 A 50-year-old man presents with progressive burning pains in the sole of his left foot, bilateral cramps in both calves and left foot drop. He is a known asthmatic and suffers from recurrent sinusitis. Full blood count shows eosinophilia.

383 A 33-year-old man presents with breathlessness at rest, cough and haemoptysis, all of which he has had for a few days. On examination he is cyanosed and there are bilateral inspiratory and expiratory wheezes. His peak flow rate is normal. Blood investigations show evidence of renal failure.

384 A 73-year-old man presents with pneumonia which he has had for 2 weeks and which has been resistant to antibiotics. He has had asthmatic bronchitis for more than 50 years. Chest radiography shows consolidation of the right upper zone and the left perihilar consolidation. Blood tests show neutrophilia.

385 A 29-year-old farmer presents with worsening cough, breathlessness and flu-like symptoms, which he has had each winter for 3 years. Chest radiography showed fine miliary shadows. Pulmonary function tests showed evidence of restrictive lung disease.

386 A 33-year-old woman presents with worsening breathlessness and dry cough. On examination there is clubbing, dyspnoea, central cyanosis, fine crepitations over the lung bases and accentuated second heart sound.

387 A 61-year-old woman presents with shortness of breath, chest pain and a single episode of haemoptysis. She had a total hip replacement 10 days ago.

Theme: Renal impairment

Options

A. Renal vein thrombosis
B. Medullary cystic disease
C. Bartter's syndrome
D. Berger's disease
E. Renal tubular acidosis
F. Nephrotic syndrome
G. Alport syndrome
H. Cystinuria
I. Renal artery stenosis
J. Rhabdomyolysis
K. Fanconi's syndrome

Instructions

For each case, choose the single most appropriate diagnosis from the list of options above. Each option may be used once, more than once or not at all.

388 A 10-year-old boy presents with nocturnal enuresis, easy fatiguability and poor progress at school. On examination he looks short and is normotensive. Blood tests show hypokalaemic hypochloraemic alkalosis.

389 A 62-year-old epileptic was found unconscious at home. Blood tests showed evidence of renal failure. Urine dipstick shows blood +++. Ammonium sulphate test shows coloured supernatant.

390 A 12-year-old girl presents with marked oedema. Blood tests show hypoalbuminaemia. Urine shows heavy proteinuria.

391 A 16-year-old student presents with a 4-month history of urinary frequency. Examination showed no abnormalities, apart from a mild hearing impairment. Blood tests showed evidence of mild renal impairment.

392 A 35-year-old man presents with acute abdominal pain. He had been fit until a month ago, when he noticed increasing swelling of both legs, up to his pelvis. Chest examination showed dullness at the right base with decreased air entry. Abdominal examination showed tenderness at the right iliac fossa. His blood tests showed evidence of renal failure.

393 A 40-year-old insurance broker presents with backache and pelvic pain. Radiography of the spine showed osteoporotic changes and medullary calcification of the kidney.

Theme: Investigating infertility

Options

    A. Vaginal wall smear
    B. Post-coital test
    C. Temperature chart
    D. Hysterosalpingography
    E. Plasma progesterone
    F. Semen analysis
    G. Endometrial biopsy
    H. Cervical mucus studies
    I. Laparoscopy
    J. Tubal insufflation
    K. Chlamydia testing

Instructions

For each statement, choose the single most appropriate investigation from the list of options above. Each option may be used once, more than once or not at all.

394 Assessment of the quantity and quality of cervical mucus and sperm interaction. B

395 Detection of intrauterine malformation and pathology. D

396 Detection of endometriosis, swellings or adhesions. I

397 Investigating a young female with dysuria, vaginal discharge and pelvic pain. K

398 A fern-like pattern is seen in the preovulatory phase but not in the post-ovulatory phase. H

Theme: Teratogenic infections during pregnancy

Options

- A. Coxsackie B virus
- B. Varicella zoster virus
- C. Cytomegalovirus
- D. Herpes simplex virus hominis type 2
- E. Toxoplasmosis
- F. Mumps
- G. Hepatitis A
- H. Syphilis
- I. Malaria
- J. Rubella virus

Instructions

For each item, choose the single most appropriate infection from the list of options above. Each option may be used once, more than once or not at all.

399 Only very rarely leads to congenital infection before 16 weeks' gestation but is known to infect all infants born to women with recent infection.

400 Causes birth defects when a mother is infected with a primary infection as opposed to a recurrent infection.

401 Surviving infants may exhibit cardiac malformation, hepatitis, pancreatitis or adrenal necrosis.

402 Surviving infants may suffer from microcephaly, persistent patent ductus arteriosus, pulmonary artery stenosis, atrial septal defect, cataract or microphthalmia.

403 The characteristic triad of abnormalities includes chorioretinitis, microcephaly and cerebral calcifications.

404 Not strictly teratogenic, but infants may suffer from endocardial fibroelastosis, urogenital abnormalities, and ear and eye malformations.

Theme: Thyroid disorders

Options

- A. Thyroglossal cyst
- B. De Quervain's thyroiditis
- C. Hypothyroidism
- D. Multiple endocrine neoplasia (MEN) type 1
- E. Simple goitre
- F. Hashimoto's thyroiditis
- G. Graves' disease
- H. Multiple endocrine neoplasia (MEN) type 2
- I. Papillary carcinoma
- J. Lymphoma
- K. Follicular carcinoma

Instructions

For each case, choose the single most appropriate diagnosis from the list of options above. Each option may be used once, more than once or not at all.

405 A 27-year-old woman presents with fever, sore throat and dysphagia. On examination she has a fine tremor and a diffusely tender thyroid. Radioisotope scan shows no uptake.

406 A 43-year-old woman presents with weight loss despite a good appetite, constipation, frontal headaches and metrorrhagia. She also complains of recurrent dyspepsia and peptic ulcers. Her abdominal radiography shows abdominal stones.

407 A 30-year-old woman presents with weight gain, constipation, lethargy and a flaky rash.

408 A 37-year-old woman presents with weight loss, muscle weakness, oligomenorrhoea, diarrhoea and blurring of vision. On examination there is exophthalmos and proximal myopathy.

409 A 19-year-old student presents with a neck swelling. On examination the swelling moves up with swallowing and protrusion of the tongue.

410 A 49-year-old woman presents with goitre. On examination the thyroid is firm and rubbery. Thyroid microsomal antibodies are positive in high titre.

Theme: Infections

Options

- A. Tuberculosis
- B. Lyme disease
- C. Toxic shock syndrome
- D. Salmonellosis
- E. Trichinosis
- F. Bacillary dysentery
- G. Leptospirosis (Weil's disease)
- H. Toxoplasmosis
- I. Amoebic hepatitis
- J. Visceral leishmaniasis
- K. Actinomycosis

Instructions

For each case, choose the single most appropriate infection from the list of options above. Each option may be used once, more than once or not at all.

411 A 30-year-old HIV-positive man developed fits. On examination there were generalised lymphadenopathy, tender nodules on his legs, right homonymous hemianopia and mild right pyramidal weakness. CT showed a right frontoparietal space-occupying lesion.

412 A 29-year-old photographer presents with diplopia. He has a past history of facial palsy and recurrent knee swelling. On examination there was mild meningism and partial left III palsy. There was no evidence of residual VII palsy. Both knees were swollen and tender. There were increased protein and white blood cells in the cerebrospinal fluid.

413 A 19-year-old student presents with acute diplopia, fever and tongue pain. He had had an episode of gastroenteritis during a trip to Alaska 2 weeks earlier. On examination there was facial swelling and subconjunctival haemorrhage in addition to bilateral ophthalmoplegia. Tongue movements were weak bilaterally. The rest of the examination was normal.

414 A 42-year-old Asian immigrant presents with a 2-month history of fever and weight loss. On examination there was generalised lymphadenopathy, hepatomegaly and huge splenomegaly. His ankles were swollen but there was no evidence of chronic liver disease.

415 A 27-year-old abattoir worker presents with myalgia and jaundice. On examination his conjunctivae were injected and there was diffuse petechial rash. There was no organomegaly.

416 A 23-year-old woman was admitted with diarrhoea, fever and headache. She was menstruating for 3 days prior to admission. On examination she is confused and flushed and there is a macular rash and bilateral conjunctivitis. Her pulse is 120 bpm and her blood pressure is 88/64 mmHg.

Theme: Gastrointestinal disorders

Options

- A. Submandibular gland stones (submandibular sialolithiasis)
- B. Oesophageal cancer
- C. Gastric carcinoma
- D. Cardiac achalasia
- E. Hiatus hernia
- F. Gastric ulcer
- G. Volvulus
- H. Intussusception
- I. Pharyngeal pouch (Zenker's diverticulum)
- J. Appendicitis
- K. Parotid gland stones (parotid sialolithiasis)
- L. Acute diverticulitis

Instructions

For each case, choose the single most appropriate diagnosis from the list of options above. Each option may be used once, more than once or not at all.

417 A 70-year-old alcoholic and heavy smoker presents with a 3-month history of progressive dysphagia and weight loss.

418 A 78-year-old man presents with a 2-week history of dysphagia where the first mouthful is swallowed easily, followed by difficulty swallowing further food and a sensation of a neck lump. He also noted halitosis and occasional food regurgitation.

419 A 53-year-old woman presents with acute severe pain triggered by eating or chewing food, associated with a swelling in the left submandibular region.

420 A 57-year-old man with an 8-week history of dysphagia undergoes a barium swallow. It shows a bird's beak deformity of the distal oesophagus with proximal dilatation.

421 A 69-year-old man with a long history of constipation presents with a 2-day history of worsening left lower quadrant abdominal pain. On examination he is pyrexial and there is tenderness in the left iliac fossa. Full blood count shows leucocytosis.

Theme: Management of myasthenia gravis

Options

- A. Corticosteroids
- B. Radiotherapy and chemotherapy
- C. Partial thymectomy
- D. Thymectomy and radiotherapy
- E. Thymectomy
- F. Expectant management
- G. Anticholinesterases
- H. Azathioprine
- I. Radiotherapy
- J. Chemotherapy
- K. Plasmapheresis and/or IV immunoglobulins

Instructions

For each case, choose the single most appropriate management from the list of options above. Each option may be used once, more than once or not at all.

422 A 40-year-old man with malignant thymoma.

423 A 49-year-old woman with generalised myasthenia gravis and a benign thymoma.

424 A 42-year-old woman with ocular myasthenia gravis and a normal thymus gland.

425 A 32-year-old woman recently diagnosed with myasthenia gravis and a benign thymoma.

426 A 30-year-old woman presents with acute myasthaenic crisis.

Theme: Rheumatology

Options

    A. Scleroderma
    B. Giant cell arteritis
    C. Ankylosing spondylitis
    D. Polymyositis
    E. CREST syndrome
    F. Systemic lupus erythematosus
    G. Polyarteritis nodosa
    H. Rheumatoid arthritis
    I. Reiter's syndrome
    J. Antiphospholipid syndrome
    K. Sjögren's syndrome

Instructions

For each case, choose the single most appropriate diagnosis from the list of options above. Each option may be used once, more than once or not at all.

427 A 38-year-old man presents with progressive breathlessness, unproductive cough and difficulty in swallowing. He also noted that his hands become painful and pale in cold weather. Chest radiographs showed patchy shadows in both mid-zones and bases. Radiography of the hands showed calcification.

428 A 31-year-old travel agent presents with painful knees, red eyes and dysuria. He has just returned from a trip to Spain.

429 A 78-year-old woman presents with headache, anorexia and fever which she has had for a few weeks. Erythrocyte sedimentation rate (ESR), C-reactive protein (CRP) and platelets were elevated, while haemoglobin was low.

430 A 36-year-old woman complains of recurrent chest pain, which is worse on inspiration, and progressive breathlessness. She also suffers from Raynaud's phenomenon. On examination she has a butterfly rash, and a pericardial rub is audible.

431 A 45-year-old woman presents with a 4-month history of multiple joint pain and progressive difficulty climbing stairs. Muscle biopsy was normal. EMG showed spontaneous fibrillation, high-frequency repetitive potentials and polyphasic potentials on voluntary contractions.

432 A 46-year-old woman complains of dryness of the mouth and eyes, joint pain and difficulty in swallowing. Schirmer's test and Rose Bengal staining are both positive.

Theme: Sexually transmitted diseases

Options
- A. Syphilis
- B. Gonorrhoea
- C. AIDS
- D. Lymphogranuloma venereum
- E. Chancroid
- F. *Molluscum contagiosum*
- G. Herpes simplex virus type 2
- H. *Gardnerella vaginalis*
- I. *Chlamydia trachomatis*
- J. Trichomoniasis
- K. Candidiasis

Instructions

For each case, choose the single most appropriate diagnosis from the list of options above. Each option may be used once, more than once or not at all.

433 A 23-year-old man presents with dysuria, urethral discharge and joint pain. Gram staining shows Gram-negative intracellular diplococci.

434 A 27-year-old African immigrant presents with painful fixed inguinal lymphadenopathy. Three weeks earlier he had had a painless papule on his genitalia which ulcerated, then healed.

435 A 31-year-old woman presents with fever, myalgia, headache and multiple painful shallow ulcers in the vulva. On examination there are also ulcers in the cervix and tender inguinal lymphadenopathy. Four weeks after treatment and recovery her symptoms recur but are less severe.

436 A 37-year-old multipara presents with vaginal discharge. Ten days earlier she had used a medication for yeast infection. She also complains of a strong odour after intercourse.

437 A 20-year-old married woman presents with a 2-week history of sporadic lower abdominal pain accompanied by a low-grade fever. She also reports an increasing amount of cloudy, non-irritating discharge and dysuria.

438 A 25-year-old sexually active woman presents with vaginal itching and discomfort that increases during intercourse and urination. She also noted greenish frothy foul-smelling vaginal discharge.

Theme: Adverse effects of medications

Options
- A. Danazol
- B. Clomiphene citrate
- C. Methotrexate
- D. GnRH analogues
- E. Oxytocin
- F. Bromocriptine
- G. Progestogens
- H. Hormone replacement therapy
- I. Prednisolone
- J. Non-steroidal anti-inflammatory drugs

Instructions

For each set of adverse effects, choose the single most appropriate causative medication from the list of options above. Each option may be used once, more than once or not at all.

439 Weight gain, acne, growth of facial hair, voice changes, decreased breast size, atrophic vaginitis and dyspareunia.

440 Osteoporosis in cases of prolonged use, hot flushes, decreased libido and vaginal dryness.

441 Breakthrough bleeding, weight gain, depression, prolonged amenorrhoea after starting treatment.

442 Visual disturbances, ovarian hyperstimulation, hot flushes, headache, weight gain, depression and abdominal discomfort.

443 May increase the risk of breast cancer and deep venous thrombosis. Side effects include weight gain, abdominal discomfort, depression and jaundice.

444 Headache, postural hypotension and Raynaud's phenomenon. High doses may cause retroperitoneal fibrosis.

Theme: Breast lumps

Options

A. Fibroadenoma
B. Breast abscess
C. Fibroadenosis
D. Breast cyst
E. Invasive ductal carcinoma
F. Fat necrosis
G. Radial scar
H. Lipoma
I. Duct ectasia
J. Intraductal papilloma
K. Paget's disease of the nipple

Instructions

For each case, choose the single most appropriate diagnosis from the list of options above. Each option may be used once, more than once or not at all.

445 A 28-year-old woman presents with a tender mass in the lower outer quadrant of the right breast, 3 weeks after giving birth. On examination overlying skin is red, hot and tender, and her temperature is 38°C.

446 A 54-year-old woman presents with a 2-week history of creamy discharge from the left nipple. On examination there is a poorly defined subareolar mass. Breast ultrasound scan shows subareolar duct dilatation.

447 A 39-year-old woman presents with a mass in the right breast that feels larger and more tender during the second half of the menstrual cycle.

448 A 60-year-old woman presents with a hard lump in the lower inner quadrant of the right breast. On examination axillary lymphadenopathy is palpable. Mammography showed a 2.5-cm mass with microcalcification.

449 A 25-year-old woman presents with a 3-cm mass in the outer upper quadrant of the left breast. On examination the mass is mobile. Ultrasound reveals that the mass is solid, with well-defined margins. FNAC shows no malignant cells.

Theme: Malabsorption

Options

A. Chronic pancreatitis
B. Crohn's disease
C. Cystic fibrosis
D. Intestinal lymphangiectasia
E. Immunodeficiency
F. Pancreatic carcinoma
G. Coeliac disease
H. Whipple's disease
I. Thyrotoxicosis
J. Post-infectious malabsorption
K. Obstructive jaundice

Instructions

For each case, choose the single most appropriate diagnosis from the list of options above. Each option may be used once, more than once or not at all.

450 A 38-year-old man presents with recurrent arthritis, diarrhoea and steatorrhoea. On examination there were bilateral small knee effusions. Small bowel biopsy showed periodic acid Schiff (PAS)-positive material in the lamina propria.

451 A 50-year-old architect presents with a 1-year history of lethargy, weight loss, diarrhoea and low back pain. On examination there was evidence of proximal myopathy and mild pitting oedema. Faecal fat excretion was increased.

452 A 65-year-old man presents with severe epigastric pain and weight loss. The pain is severe and radiating to the back. On examination there is a palpable epigastric mass and hepatomegaly.

453 A 38-year-old man presents with bloody diarrhoea, abdominal discomfort and weight loss. On examination there is a tender palpable mass in the right iliac fossa.

454 A 16-year-old student presents with abdominal pain and diarrhoea. She has had recurrent chest infections for most of her life.

455 A 58-year-old alcoholic complains of epigastric pain of 5 months' duration. The pain gets worse after heavy alcohol consumption. He also complains of diarrhoea and weight loss. Abdominal radiography shows multiple calcifications.

Theme: Congenital cardiac lesions

Options

A. Atrial septal defect
B. Ebstein's anomaly
C. Congenital pulmonary stenosis
D. Ventricular septal defect
E. Patent ductus arteriosus
F. Hypertrophic obstructive cardiomyopathy
G. Fallot's tetralogy
H. Coarctation of the aorta and bicuspid aortic valve
I. Dextrocardia
J. Transposition of the great arteries
K. Congenital aortic stenosis

Instructions

For each case, choose the single most appropriate diagnosis from the list of options above. Each option may be used once, more than once or not at all.

456 A 27-year-old woman presents with headache. On examination her blood pressure was 165/115 mmHg, pulse was 90 bpm, and there was an ejection click in the aortic area and an ejection systolic murmur all over the precordium and back.

457 A 39-year-old man presents with progressive breathlessness and palpitations. On examination the JVP was elevated with a prominent 'a' wave and there was a pulmonary ejection systolic murmur. ECG showed a right bundle branch block with large P waves.

458 A 3-year-old boy with a history of recurrent chest infections presents with worsening shortness of breath. On examination there was systolic thrill at the left lower sternal edge, pansystolic murmur and accentuated second heart sound.

459 A 21-year-old man presents with worsening shortness of breath. He had been told that he had had a murmur since he was a child. On examination there was a continuous murmur and the pulse was bounding.

460 A 5-year-old boy was referred for poor growth and worsening shortness of breath. On examination he was cyanosed and there was clubbing. There was an ejection systolic murmur, single second heart sound and a parasternal heave. Chest radiography showed right ventricular hypertrophy and a small pulmonary artery.

461 An infant was referred for heart failure and cyanosis. On examination there was elevated JVP, hepatomegaly, pansystolic murmur at the lower left sternal edge and third heart sound. Chest radiography showed a large globular heart. ECG showed right bundle branch block.

Theme: Management of gastrointestinal disorders

Options

    A. CT of the abdomen
    B. Oesophageal manometry
    C. Motility studies
    D. Mesenteric angiography
    E. Percutaneous transhepatic cholangiogram
    F. Barium enema
    G. Upper gastrointestinal endoscopy
    H. Barium meal
    I. Ultrasound scan
    J. Erect and supine abdominal radiography

Instructions

For each case, choose the single most appropriate investigation from the list of options above. Each option may be used once, more than once or not at all.

462 A 49-year-old alcoholic presents with haematemesis and melaena. He is stable after being transfused two units of blood.

463 A 56-year-old man presents with massive persistent fresh rectal bleeding. A recent barium enema showed no evidence of diverticulosis or tumours. Nasogastric suction showed yellow bile and no evidence of bleeding.

464 A 59-year-old man presents with a 2-day history of worsening crampy abdominal pain, constipation and recurrent vomiting. On examination his abdomen is distended, with high-pitched bowel sounds. There is no localised tenderness or rectal mass.

465 A 65-year-old woman presents with a 1-year history of pain in the right upper quadrant exacerbated by eating rich foods.

466 A 68-year-old man presents with obstructive jaundice and severe weight loss of 2 months' duration. Abdominal ultrasonography shows a 5-cm mass with dilated bile ducts in the head of the pancreas.

Theme: Blood supply to the brain

Options
- A. Basilar artery
- B. Anterior cerebral artery
- C. Superior cerebellar artery
- D. Posterior cerebral artery
- E. Anterior communicating artery
- F. Middle cerebral artery
- G. Circle of Willis
- H. Posterior communicating artery
- I. Anterior inferior cerebellar artery
- J. Anterior spinal artery
- K. Posterior inferior cerebellar artery

Instructions

For each area of the brain, choose the single most appropriate blood supply from the list of options above. Each option may be used once, more than once or not at all.

467 Broca's area of speech
468 Trigeminal nerve nucleus in the medulla oblongata
469 Visual cortex
470 Leg area in the motor cortex
471 Anterior aspect of the pons
472 Arm and face areas in the motor cortex

Theme: Chest pain in pregnancy

Options

- A. Aortic dissection
- B. Massive pulmonary embolism
- C. Pulmonary infarction
- D. Myocardial infarction
- E. Aortic rupture
- F. Hysteria
- G. Pneumothorax
- H. Oesophageal spasm
- I. Pericarditis
- J. Musculoskeletal pain

Instructions

For each case, choose the single most appropriate diagnosis from the list of options above. Each option may be used once, more than once or not at all.

473 A 30-year-old pregnant woman (31 weeks) presents with severe chest pain of acute onset. There is a family history of ischaemic heart disease (IHD). Clinical examination demonstrates dyspnoea, cyanosis, hypotension (90/50 mmHg) and distended neck veins.

474 A 25-year-old pregnant woman (24 weeks) presents with a 3-day history of bilateral chest pain. She has suffered from a dry cough for a week. On examination her chest is clear, but there are multiple points of tenderness over the chest wall.

475 A tall, slim 30-year-old pregnant woman (26 weeks) presents with central chest pain. General examination reveals arachnodactyly and scoliosis, while her blood pressure is 90/40 mmHg and her pulse is 116 bpm.

476 A 33-year-old pregnant woman (29 weeks) presents with inspiratory chest pain. The pain is much less when she sits up and leans forward. She had an upper respiratory tract infection a week earlier.

Theme: Blood film

Options

A. Infectious mononucleosis
B. Iron deficiency anaemia
C. Malaria
D. Thrombotic thrombocytopenic purpura
E. Megaloblastic anaemia
F. Sickle cell disease
G. Multiple myeloma
H. Acute myeloid leukaemia
I. Myelofibrosis
J. β-thalassaemia major
K. Chronic lymphatic leukaemia

Instructions

For each blood film, choose the single most appropriate diagnosis from the list of options above. Each option may be used once, more than once or not at all.

477 Hypochromic microcytic red cells and cigar-shaped cells.

478 Poikilocytosis, anisocytosis, macrocytosis, teardrop cells and hyper-segmented polymorphs. The macrocytes are oval rather than round.

479 Microcytosis, anisocytosis, poikilocytosis, hypochromia, target cells and teardrop cells.

480 Sickle cells, target cells and nucleated red cells.

481 Leucoerythroblastic blood film with immature white cells and nucleated red cells, anisocytosis, poikilocytosis and teardrop cells.

482 Stacking of red cells into rouleaux and abnormal plasma cells.

Theme: Arthritis

Options

A. Systemic lupus erythematosus
B. Antiphospholipid syndrome
C. Reiter's syndrome
D. Rheumatoid arthritis
E. Felty's syndrome
F. Giant cell arteritis
G. Sjögren's syndrome
H. Scleroderma
I. Polyarteritis nodosa
J. Osteoarthritis
K. Pseudogout

Instructions

For each case, choose the single most appropriate diagnosis from the list of options above. Each option may be used once, more than once or not at all.

483 A 53-year-old woman complains of pain, swelling and stiffness in the distal interphalangeal joints of her hands, but has no other joint complaints.

484 A 60-year-old previously fit man presents with a 2-month history of fatigue, weight loss of 5 kg, dyspnoea on exertion, abdominal pain and progressive numbness in his feet. He had recently developed mild polyarthritis in his hands. On examination there was evidence of left median nerve mononeuritis and his blood pressure was 150/100 mmHg. Chest radiography showed cardiomegaly.

485 A 79-year-old man complains of pain and swelling of the right knee. He has bilateral swollen wrists, metacarpophalangeal (MCP), proximal interphalangeal (PIP) and distal phalangeal (DIP) joints. His knee is also swollen with limitation of range of motion by pain. Radiography shows calcification of the meniscal cartilage of the knee.

486 A 22-year-old woman presents with a 3-week history of fever, pleuritic chest pain, stiffness and swelling in the wrists, MCP joints and PIP joints. On examination there is bilateral pretibial oedema.

487 A 27-year-old man presents with low back pain, pain in the right knee and sore eyes. He had had an episode of diarrhoea 3 weeks earlier, and has a positive family history of back pain. Pelvic radiography showed sclerosis and erosion of the lower joint margins.

488 A 77-year-old woman with long-standing rheumatoid arthritis presents with fever and dysuria. Her past history included recurrent chest and urinary infections. On examination she was hyperpigmented and emaciated. Her hands and feet were severely deformed. Abdominal examination revealed splenomegaly, but no hepatomegaly or lymphadenopathy.

Theme: Electrolyte imbalance

Options

    A. Primary hyperparathyroidism
    B. Addison's disease
    C. Hyperthyroidism
    D. Small cell (oat cell) carcinoma
    E. Cushing's disease
    F. Diabetes mellitus
    G. Diabetes insipidus
    H. Pyloric stenosis
    I. Psychogenic polydipsia
    J. Multiple myeloma
    K. Vitamin D deficiency

Instructions

For each biochemical profile, choose the single most appropriate diagnosis from the list of options above. Each option may be used once, more than once or not at all.

489 Hyponatraemia, hyperkalaemia, hypoglycaemia and increased urea.

490 Hyponatraemia, hypokalaemia and metabolic alkalosis.

491 Hypernatraemia, hypokalaemia and hyperglycaemia.

492 Hypoalbuminaemia, hypercalcaemia and hyperuricaemia.

493 Hyponatraemia, hypokalaemia and hypercalcaemia.

494 Hypercalcaemia, hypophosphataemia and increased alkaline phosphatase.

Theme: Dermatomes

Options

    A. C8
    B. T7
    C. L4
    D. S3
    E. T1
    F. L5
    G. T10
    H. C2
    I. S1
    J. L5
    K. C4

Instructions

For each dermatome, choose the single most appropriate nerve root from the list of options above. Each option may be used once, more than once or not at all.

495 The big toe and the anteromedial aspect of the leg.

496 The little finger and the medial aspect of the palm and dorsum of the hand.

497 The little toe and the posterolateral aspect of the heel.

498 A transverse band crossing the umbilicus.

499 The medial aspect of the arm and forearm.

500 The middle three toes and the lateral aspect of the front of the leg.

Theme: Cranial nerves

Options

A. I
B. II
C. III
D. IV
E. V
F. VI
G. VII
H. VIII
I. IX
J. X
K. XI
L. XII

Instructions

For each nerve supply, choose the single most appropriate cranial nerve from the list of options above. Each option may be used once, more than once or not at all.

501 Motor fibres to the trapezius and sternomastoid.

502 Motor fibres to the muscles of the tongue.

503 Sensory fibres to the tonsillar fossa and pharynx plus taste fibres to the posterior third of the tongue.

504 Motor fibres to the muscles of mastication.

505 Motor fibres to the superior oblique muscle.

506 Motor fibres to the lateral rectus muscle.

Theme: Clinical features of AIDS

Options

A. Painful feet
B. Erythematous to violaceous cutaneous lesions with several morphologies: macular, patch, plaque or nodular.
C. Acute focal neurological deficit and seizures
D. Progressive visual impairment
E. Paralysis, loss of vision, impaired speech and cognitive deterioration
F. Acute delirium
G. Proximal muscle weakness
H. Fasciculation
I. Progressive hemiparesis impairment
J. Impotence

Instructions

For each diagnosis, choose the single most appropriate clinical feature from the list of options above. Each option may be used once, more than once or not at all.

507 Cryptococcal meningitis
508 Kaposi's sarcoma
509 Progressive multifocal leucoencephalopathy
510 Central nervous system lymphoma
511 Chronic sensory polyneuropathy
512 Cerebral toxoplasmosis

Theme: Physical signs of cardiac lesions

Options

- A. Aortic regurgitation
- B. Hypertrophic cardiomyopathy
- C. Patent ductus arteriosus
- D. Aortic stenosis
- E. Atrial septal defect
- F. Tricuspid regurgitation
- G. Mitral valve prolapse
- H. Coarctation of the aorta
- I. Mitral stenosis
- J. Ventricular septal defect
- K. Transposition of the great arteries

Instructions

For each physical sign, choose the single most appropriate diagnosis from the list of options above. Each option may be used once, more than once or not at all.

513 Pulsatile liver

514 Positive Hill's sign

515 A mid-systolic click, followed by a late systolic murmur heard best at the apex.

516 Soft, single second heart sound

517 Loud first heart sound

518 Cardiac apex is double in character.

Theme: Haematological diseases

Options

A. Paroxysmal nocturnal haemoglobinuria
B. Thrombotic thrombocytopenic purpura
C. Protein C deficiency
D. Sickle cell anaemia
E. Antiphospholipid syndrome
F. Disseminated intravascular coagulopathy
G. Polycythaemia rubra vera
H. Trousseau syndrome
I. Waldenström's macroglobulinaemia
J. Multiple myeloma
K. Myelofibrosis

Instructions

For each case, choose the single most appropriate diagnosis from the list of options above. Each option may be used once, more than once or not at all.

519 A 65-year-old woman with mitral stenosis presents with painful red lesions on her left leg and chest, 4 days after starting warfarin.

520 A 62-year-old male smoker presents with symptoms of deep venous thrombosis in the left leg and the right forearm. One month ago, he was referred to the chest physicians for management of persistent cough and haemoptysis.

521 A 29-year-old woman presents with deep venous thrombosis of the left calf. Her past history included recurrent abortions and arthritis.

522 A 42-year-old man presents with portal vein thrombosis. He has had a 4-year history of chronic iron deficiency anaemia with unknown source of blood loss.

523 A 31-year-old woman presents with vaginal bleeding 6 days after an abortion. Two hours after admission, she started fitting then lapsed into a coma. On examination her temperature was 38.3°C and pulse was 138 bpm. Blood tests showed anaemia, thrombocytopenia and a normal clotting profile. Renal function was markedly impaired.

524 A 75-year-old woman presents with headache, visual floaters, weight loss, lethargy and recurrent epistaxis. On examination she was pale with generalised lymphadenopathy and hepatosplenomegaly. Fundal examination showed right retinal vein thrombosis.

Theme: Diarrhoea

Options

A. Viral gastroenteritis
B. Ulcerative colitis
C. Coeliac disease
D. Laxative abuse
E. Thyrotoxicosis
F. *Campylobacter* infection
G. Pseudomembranous colitis
H. *Giardia lamblia* infestation
I. Collagenous colitis
J. Irritable bowel syndrome
K. Chronic pancreatitis

Instructions

For each case, choose the single most appropriate diagnosis from the list of options above. Each option may be used once, more than once or not at all.

525 A 52-year-old woman presents with a 4-year history of recurrent non-bloody diarrhoea. All investigations were normal (including radiography and endoscopy) apart from elevated ESR and colonic biopsy which showed an eosinophilic band in the subepithelial layer.

526 A previously fit 22-year-old man presents with acute bloody diarrhoea, crampy abdominal pain and low-grade fever. His symptoms resolved spontaneously in 6 days and never recurred.

527 A 28-year-old woman presents with chronic watery diarrhoea. The stools showed a positive osmotic gap. Her diarrhoea stopped within 3 days after admission and fasting.

528 A previously healthy 21-year-old man presents with a 6-week history of bloody diarrhoea, crampy abdominal pain and fever. Proctosigmoidoscopy showed bleeding and friable colonic mucosa.

529 A 27-year-old woman developed severe water diarrhoea 12 days after starting antibiotics for pelvic inflammatory disease. Proctosigmoidoscopy showed plaque-like lesions.

530 An anxious 28-year-old sales assistant presents with a 4-month history of diarrhoea alternating with constipation. The stools were usually soft and there was no history of bleeding. No abnormality was found on examination. All investigations, including flexible fibre-sigmoidoscopy and radiography, were normal.

Theme: Thyroid function tests

Options

- A. Non-toxic goitre
- B. Hashimoto's thyroiditis
- C. Subacute thyroiditis
- D. Anaplastic carcinoma
- E. Nephrotic syndrome
- F. Pregnancy
- G. Hypothyroidism
- H. Thyroid binding globulin deficiency
- I. Riedel's thyroiditis
- J. Graves' disease

Instructions

For each biochemical profile, choose the single most appropriate diagnosis from the list of options above. Each option may be used once, more than once or not at all.

531 Elevated serum T_4 and increased radioactive iodine uptake.

532 Elevated serum T_4 and low radioactive iodine uptake.

533 Elevated serum T_4 and low T_3 resin uptake.

534 Decreased serum T_4 and low T_3 resin uptake.

535 Normal serum T_3 and T_4 in a patient with a neck mass.

536 Normal serum TSH, free T_4 and T_3 with decreased serum total T_4.

Theme: Rheumatology

Options

A. Rheumatoid arthritis
B. CREST syndrome
C. Reiter's syndrome
D. Sjögren's syndrome
E. Dermatomyositis
F. Systemic lupus erythematosus
G. Polymyalgia rheumatica
H. Polymyositis
I. Giant cell arteritis
J. Takayasu's arteritis
K. Churg–Strauss syndrome
L. Antiphospholipid syndrome

Instructions

For each case, choose the single most appropriate diagnosis from the list of options above. Each option may be used once, more than once or not at all.

537 A 52-year-old woman complains of a 4-month history of Raynaud's phenomenon, progressive skin tightness, thickening of the fingers and hands, dyspnoea on exertion and dysphagia.

538 A 22-year-old woman complains of loss of appetite, low-grade fever, shoulder and buttock pains, and severe cramps in her arms and hands during exercise. On examination her pulse is weak in both arms, her blood pressure is 75/55 mmHg in the left arm, 60/40 mmHg in the right arm and 125/75 mmHg in both legs.

539 A 52-year-old man complains of a gritty sensation in his eyes and dry mouth. He also complains of arthralgia in both hands and knees. On examination there are multiple purpuric lesions over both calves and ankles.

540 A 32-year-old man presents with a rash on his penis, pain in the left heel and right-side stiffness in the lower back upon arising in the morning. Two weeks earlier, he had had an episode of diarrhoea.

541 A 73-year-old man presents with persistent malaise, anorexia, pain in the shoulders and hips, and loss of 10 kg over the last 10 weeks. On examination there is mild painful limitation of hip and shoulder motion and muscle tenderness but no weakness.

542 A 25-year-old woman presents with deep venous thrombosis in the right leg. Her past history includes three miscarriages. Her blood tests show mild thrombocytopenia and a positive serology test for syphilis.

Theme: Physical signs of congenital heart diseases

Options

A. Patent ductus arteriosus
B. Atrial septal defect
C. Aortic stenosis
D. Ebstein's anomaly
E. Ventricular septal defect
F. Pulmonary stenosis
G. Coarctation of the aorta
H. Fallot's tetralogy
I. L-transposition of the great arteries
J. Eisenmenger's syndrome
K. D-transposition of the great arteries

Instructions

For each of the following physical findings, choose the single most appropriate diagnosis from the list of options above. Each option may be used once, more than once or not at all.

543 Continuous murmur
544 Absent femoral pulses
545 Fixed, widely split second heart sound.
546 Harsh pansystolic murmur best heard at the lower left sternal border.
547 Wide splitting of the first and second heart sounds.
548 Right ventricular heave, single second heart sound and a harsh systolic ejection murmur along the sternal border.

Theme: Management of thoracic disorders

Options

A. Chest tube insertion
B. Pericardiocentesis
C. Ventilation/perfusion scan
D. Lung function tests
E. CT of the chest
F. Echocardiography
G. MRI of the chest
H. Thoracotomy and decortication
I. Local wound exploration
J. Antibiotics

Instructions

For each case, choose the single most appropriate management from the list of options above. Each option may be used once, more than once or not at all.

549 A 42-year-old man is brought to A&E with a stab wound to the right chest in the third intercostal space in the anterior axillary line. He is hypotensive and complains of shortness of breath. On examination breath sounds are absent on the right side of the chest.

550 A 57-year-old man is brought to A&E after a road traffic accident. He is conscious and stable but has severe bruising of the anterior chest. His chest radiograph shows widened mediastinum and a small left pleural effusion.

551 A 67-year-old alcoholic presents with a 2-week history of fever and purulent expectoration. Chest radiography shows an air–fluid level in the upper lobe of his left lung.

552 A 60-year-old smoker presents with haemoptysis. His chest radiograph shows a 2-cm non-calcified lesion of the upper lobe of the left lung. A radiograph taken 4 years earlier was normal.

Theme: Renal pathology

Options

    A. Wegener's granulomatosis
    B. Goodpasture's syndrome
    C. Lupus nephritis
    D. Alport syndrome
    E. Diabetic nephropathy
    F. Berger's disease
    G. Pre-eclampsia
    H. Polycystic kidneys
    I. Chronic interstitial nephritis
    J. Renal papillary necrosis
    K. Medullary sponge kidney

Instructions

For each renal pathology, choose the single most appropriate diagnosis from the list of options above. Each option may be used once, more than once or not at all.

553 Necrotising granulomatous vasculitis

554 Nodular glomerulosclerosis

555 Focal segmental glomerulosclerosis

556 Positive fluorescent antinuclear antibody (ANA)

557 Glomerular capillary endotheliosis

558 Highly cellular crescentic proliferative glomerulonephritis

Theme: Management of cardiac patients

Options

A. Add a β-blocker
B. Add an ACE inhibitor
C. Add an angiotensin 2 blocker
D. No further action needed at this stage
E. Add spironolactone
F. Request an echo cardiogram
G. Request a 24-hour tape
H. Add furosemide
I. Check thyroid function
J. Request a renal ultrasound scan
K. Request a 24-hour blood pressure monitor

Instructions

For each case, choose the single most appropriate management from the list of options above. Each option may be used once, more than once or not at all.

559 A 50-year-old hypertensive man on an ACE inhibitor is referred to the heart failure clinic. His blood pressure is 136/86 mmHg and his pulse 92 bpm (regular rhythm). There is no evidence of fluid overload.

560 A 42-year-old man is found to have a blood pressure above 150/90 mmHg on four separate occasions. A renal ultrasound scan was normal as well as a variety of blood and urine tests.

561 A 60-year-old woman complains of intermittent palpitations lasting a few minutes, several times during the day. Her GP reviews her records and notes that she had had a normal echocardiogram 6 months earlier and a normal thyroid function test a month earlier.

562 A 69-year-old man with long-standing heart failure is reviewed because of worsening shortness of breath. He is already on maximum doses of an ACE inhibitor and a β-blocker. His blood pressure was 130/82 mmHg and his pulse was 72 bpm (regular rhythm). His renal function showed stage 2 CKD with a normal potassium level, and his echocardiogram showed a moderately impaired left ventricular systolic function.

563 A 27-year-old woman presents with a 2-month history of palpitations and weight loss. She feels that she is anxious all the time as she is under a lot of stress. Her blood pressure is 128/80 mmHg and her pulse is 96 bpm (regular rhythm).

Theme: Tumour markers

Options

- A. CA 15-3
- B. CA 125
- C. CA 19-9
- D. Carcinoembryonic antigen (CEA)
- E. α-fetoprotein (AFP)
- F. Human chorionic gonadotrophin (HCG)
- G. Calcitonin
- H. Thyroglobulin
- I. Prostate-specific antigen (PSA)
- J. S-100

Instructions

For each tumour, choose the single most appropriate tumour marker from the list of options above. Each option may be used once, more than once or not at all.

564 Medullary thyroid carcinoma

565 Hepatocellular carcinoma

566 Rectal carcinoma

567 Papillary thyroid carcinoma

568 Malignant melanoma

Theme: Neurological disorders

Options

A. Guillain–Barré syndrome
B. Labyrinthitis
C. Anterior spinal artery occlusion
D. Alzheimer's disease
E. Multiple system atrophy
F. Multiple sclerosis
G. Glioblastoma multiforme
H. Vertebral artery dissection
I. Chronic inflammatory demyelinating polyneuropathy
J. Cauda equina syndrome
K. Parkinson's disease
L. Meningioma

Instructions

For each case, choose the single most appropriate diagnosis from the list of options above. Each option may be used once, more than once or not at all.

569 A 38-year-old diver developed headache, dizziness, right hemiparesis and loss of pain and temperature sensation in the right facial and left side of the body following a dive.

570 A hypertensive 78-year-old male smoker presents after a fall. On examination there was weakness of both legs with loss of pain and temperature sensation and areflexia. His bladder was distended.

571 A 58-year-old man presents with a 10-month history of impotence and dizzy spells. On examination there was bradykinesia, rigidity, postural hypotension and tremors.

572 A 75-year-old woman presents with a 3-week history of headache and progressive confusion. On examination she had right hemianopia. CT showed a large irregularly enhancing mass in the left parietal lobe. There was no evidence of systemic disease.

573 A healthy 72-year-old woman presents with auditory hallucinations. During the interview she seemed incoherent. Examination was unremarkable.

574 A 73-year-old man presents with a 3-month history of progressive difficulty walking. On examination he had distal weakness in the arms and legs. Muscle stretch reflexes were absent. Motor nerve conduction velocities were slowed.

Theme: Vasculitis

Options
A. Microscopic polyangiitis
B. Takayasu's arteritis
C. Wegener's granulomatosis
D. Kawasaki disease
E. Henoch–Schönlein purpura
F. Churg–Strauss syndrome
G. Polyarteritis nodosa
H. Giant cell arteritis
I. Cryoglobulinaemic vasculitis
J. Goodpasture's syndrome
K. Behçet's disease

Instructions

For each case, choose the single most appropriate diagnosis from the list of options above. Each option may be used once, more than once or not at all.

575 A 22-year-old woman presents with worsening headache, nausea, painful neck and fever. A year ago she had developed pain in her legs on running. On examination her blood pressure was 190/105 mmHg, femoral pulses were weak with a radio-femoral delay and an abdominal bruit was heard.

576 A 16-year-old student presents with severe chest pain. On examination his temperature was 38.8°C, blood pressure was 100/60 mmHg and pulse was 120 bpm. There was also conjunctival congestion, polymorphous rash and palpable lymphadenopathy.

577 A 79-year-old man presents with a 24-hour history of acute loss of vision in his left eye. He had had severe temporal headaches for about 6 months. On examination the left optic disc was swollen with flame-shaped haemorrhage at 7 o'clock. Eye movements were full and painless.

578 A 28-year-old man presents with fever, myalgia and abdominal pain. On examination his temperature was 38.8°C, blood pressure was 190/110 mmHg and pulse was 120 bpm. His abdomen was tender with guarding and absent bowel sounds.

579 A 42-year-old man with a long history of asthma presents with excessive shortness of breath, weight loss, cough and occasional haemoptysis. He also complained of numbness and weakness of the left leg, which he has had for 3 months. On examination his temperature was 38.3°C and there was evidence of left sensory motor neuropathy. Full blood count showed eosinophilia. Chest radiography showed pulmonary infiltrates.

580 A 13-year-old boy was admitted with a tender swollen left knee and a tender right elbow. His past history included recurrent sore throats and dull abdominal pain for a few days. On examination his temperature was 37.9°C and there was some periumbilical tenderness. Both urine and stools were positive for blood.

Theme: Acute abdominal pain

Options

A. Acute intermittent porphyria
B. Acute pancreatitis
C. Ischaemic colitis
D. Sigmoid volvulus
E. Intussusception
F. Familial Mediterranean fever
G. Acute appendicitis
H. Paroxysmal nocturnal haemoglobinuria
I. Diverticulitis
J. Meckel's diverticulitis
K. Perforated peptic ulcer
L. Inflammatory bowel disease

Instructions

For each case, choose the single most appropriate diagnosis from the list of options above. Each option may be used once, more than once or not at all.

581 A 63-year-old man presents with vomiting, bloody diarrhoea and acute pain in the left iliac fossa. He had had a similar episode which followed a heavy meal, and he had had two myocardial infarcts over the last 10 years. On examination his temperature was 37.7°C and his left iliac fossa was tender with no guarding.

582 A 73-year-old woman presents with sudden severe left-side abdominal pain while straining to pass stools. She has a long history of constipation. On examination she was afebrile. Her abdomen was distended, particularly on the left, and tender and tympanitic with increased bowel sounds.

583 A 24-year-old Cypriot student presents with severe abdominal pain, fever and a tender swollen left knee. Four weeks ago he had also suffered from a similar swelling in his right ankle. On examination his temperature was 39°C and his abdomen was diffusely tender. Urinalysis showed protein +++, blood negative and glucose negative.

584 A 34-year-old Spanish lawyer presents with severe colicky central abdominal pain radiating to the back. She had recently been started on barbiturates for convulsions and insomnia. On examination her temperature was 38.1°C and there was a laparotomy scar with no evidence of organomegaly.

585 A 37-year-old woman presents with worsening fatigue and intermittent abdominal pain. Three weeks ago, she had had an axillary vein thrombosis. On examination she was mildly jaundiced. Full blood count showed anaemia, leucopenia and thrombocytopenia. Urine analysis was positive for blood.

586 A 2-year-old boy presents with a 6-hour history of pain in the right iliac fossa and fresh bleeding per rectum. On examination his temperature was 36.5°C, blood pressure was 100/60 mmHg and pulse was 100 bpm.

Theme: Risk factors for malignancies

Options

A. Asbestosis
B. Aniline dye
C. Hypercalcaemia
D. Pernicious anaemia
E. Early menarche and late menopause
F. Epstein–Barr virus
G. Nulliparity
H. Ulcerative colitis
I. Multiple sexual partners
J. Xeroderma pigmentosum
K. Polycystic kidney disease

Instructions

For each malignant tumour, choose the single most appropriate risk factor from the list of options above. Each option may be used once, more than once or not at all.

587 Gastric carcinoma
588 Ovarian carcinoma
589 Colorectal carcinoma
590 Bladder carcinoma
591 Lung carcinoma
592 Burkitt's lymphoma

Theme: Haematuria

Options

A. Urinary tract infection
B. Transitional cell carcinoma of the urinary bladder
C. Renal adenocarcinoma
D. Ureteric calculus
E. Prostatic carcinoma
F. Prostatic hyperplasia
G. Urinary bladder calculus
H. Haemorrhagic cystitis
I. Glomerulonephritis
J. Polycystic disease of the kidney
K. Vasculitis

Instructions

For each case, choose the single most appropriate diagnosis from the list of options above. Each option may be used once, more than once or not at all.

593 A 51-year-old man presents with a 2-month history of haematuria and pain in the right flank. Urine microscopy confirms haematuria (Hb 19 g/dL, WCC 1300/mm^3, haematocrit 59%).

594 A 20-year-old woman presents with urinary frequency, haematuria and lower abdominal pain.

595 A 75-year-old man presents with haematuria and backache. Plain radiographs show sclerotic areas in the lumbosacral spine.

596 A 56-year-old male smoker with a history of severe rheumatoid arthritis treated with cyclophosphamide presents with a 3-month history of haematuria. A plain abdominal radiograph shows two small rounded spinal lesions.

597 A 35-year-old surgeon presents with severe flank pain, nausea and vomiting. Urine microscopy shows red blood cells and crystals (Hb 14 g/dL, WCC 1500/mm^3).

Theme: Genetic disorders

Options
- A. Turner's syndrome
- B. Triple X syndrome
- C. Fragile X syndrome
- D. Down's syndrome
- E. Patau's syndrome
- F. Klinefelter's syndrome
- G. Double Y syndrome
- H. Edwards' syndrome

Instructions

For each set of clinical findings, choose the single most appropriate diagnosis from the list of options above. Each option may be used once, more than once or not at all.

598 Low-set ears, micrognathia, rocker-bottom feet and learning difficulties.

599 Low-set ears, cleft lip, microphthalmia and learning difficulties.

600 Tall, fertile male, minor mental and psychiatric illness.

601 Infertile male, testicular atrophy, gynaecomastia and learning difficulties.

602 Flat face, slanting eyes, simian crease, hypotonia and learning difficulties.

603 Primary amenorrhoea, short stature, cubitus vulgus and normal IQ.

Theme: Metabolic disturbances

Options

A. Hypokalaemia
B. Hyponatraemia
C. Hypervitaminosis A
D. Hyperkalaemia
E. Hypoglycaemia
F. Hyperglycaemia
G. Hypocalcaemia
H. Hypermagnesaemia
I. Hypernatraemia
J. Hypercalcaemia
K. Hypophosphataemia

Instructions

For each clinical presentation, choose the single most appropriate metabolic disorder from the list of options above. Each option may be used once, more than once or not at all.

604 Restlessness, confusion, irritability, seizures and coma.

605 Muscle weakness, bradycardia and hypotension. ECG shows tall peaked T waves.

606 Sweating, palpitations, tremors, drowsiness and fatigue.

607 Muscle weakness and ectopic beats. ECG shows flattened or inverted T waves.

608 Perioral paraesthesia, carpopedal spasm and generalised seizures.

609 Severe abdominal pain, nausea, vomiting, constipation, polyuria and polydipsia.

Theme: Erythropoietin level

Options

A. Polycythaemia secondary to hepatoma
B. Congenital spherocytosis
C. Polycythaemia rubra vera
D. Thalassaemia minor
E. Anaemia of chronic disease
F. Renal failure
G. Aplastic anaemia
H. Glucose-6-phosphate dehydrogenase (G6PD) deficiency
I. Von Willebrand disease
J. Haemophilia A

Instructions

For each biochemical profile, choose the single most appropriate diagnosis from the list of options above. Each option may be used once, more than once or not at all.

610 Normal or slightly elevated plasma erythropoietin with a variable response to exogenous erythropoietin.

611 Elevated plasma erythropoietin with a poor response to exogenous erythropoietin.

612 Extremely high plasma erythropoietin levels.

613 Low or absent plasma erythropoietin.

614 Low erythropoietin levels with a good response to exogenous erythropoietin.

Theme: Immunodeficiency disorders

Options
- A. DiGeorge syndrome
- B. Nezelof syndrome
- C. Wiskott–Aldrich syndrome
- D. Leucocyte adhesion deficiency
- E. Ataxia telangiectasia
- F. Severe combined immunodeficiency
- G. Bruton's agammaglobulinaemia
- H. Chédiak–Steinbrinck–Higashi syndrome
- I. Chronic granulomatous disease
- J. Job's syndrome (hyperimmunoglobulin E syndrome)
- K. Selective IgA deficiency

Instructions

For each statement below, choose the single most appropriate diagnosis from the list of options above. Each option may be used once, more than once or not at all.

615 Low lymphocyte count
616 Increased IgE and eosinophilia
617 Giant lysosomal granules in granulocytes
618 Low serum calcium level
619 Nitroblue tetrazolium test (NBT)
620 Abnormal platelet number and morphology

Theme: Investigations during pregnancy

Options
- A. Kleihauer–Betke test
- B. Liver function test
- C. Oral glucose tolerance test
- D. Amniocentesis
- E. Full blood count
- F. Abdominal ultrasound
- G. 24-hour urine protein excretion
- H. Sickling test
- I. Skin allergy test
- J. ECG
- K. Maternal DNA sampling
- L. Urine for microscopy, culture and sensitivity
- M. Chorionic villus sampling

Instructions

For each case, choose the single most appropriate investigation from the list of options above. Each option may be used once, more than once or not at all.

621 A 36-year-old para 3+1 who is 16 weeks pregnant has a triple test which shows that her baby has an increased risk of having Down's syndrome.

622 A 24-year-old primiparous woman presents at 33 weeks' gestation with itching.

623 A 23-year-old primiparous woman presents at 31 weeks' gestation with profuse vaginal bleeding. She is rhesus negative.

624 A 32-year-old para 2+1 presents at 36 weeks' gestation with a blood pressure of 175/100 mmHg and proteinuria ++.

625 A 30-year-old primiparous 35-week pregnant woman is noted to have a symphyseal-fundal height of 28 cm.

Theme: Bone profile interpretation

Options
- A. Hypoparathyroidism
- B. Pseudohypoparathyroidism
- C. Pseudopseudohypoparathyroidism
- D. Primary hyperparathyroidism
- E. Tertiary hyperparathyroidism
- F. Chronic renal failure
- G. Sarcoidosis
- H. DiGeorge syndrome
- I. Paget's disease of bone
- J. Bone metastases
- K. Osteomalacia
- L. Multiple myeloma

Instructions

For each case, choose the single most appropriate diagnosis from the list of options above. Each option may be used once, more than once or not at all.

626 A 19-year-old man presents to A&E with an epileptic fit. He is noted to have a short stature and small hands. X-ray of hands shows short fourth and fifth metacarpals. Investigations: normal renal function and glucose, Ca 1.72 mmol/L, phosphate 2.12 mmol/L and albumin 40 g/L.

627 A 47-year-old vegan presents to her GP with ache in both legs and hips. Investigations: normal full blood count, renal function and thyroid function tests; calcium 2.15 mmol/L, phosphate 0.95 mmol/L, alkaline phosphatase 480 IU/L and albumin 31 g/L.

628 A 63-year-old man presents to his GP with a 3-month history of low back pain. Investigations: Hb 8.9 g/dL, MCV 84 fL, WCC 6.7 × 10⁹/L, platelets 251 × 10⁹/L, ESR 96 mm in first hour, calcium 2.88 mmol/L, alkaline phosphatase 128 IU/L and albumin 30 g/L.

629 A 9-year-old girl is brought to A&E after a grand mal fit. X-ray shows normal hand bones. Investigations: normal renal function and glucose, calcium 1.69 mmol/L, phosphate 1.93 mmol/L, alkaline phosphatase 162 IU/L and albumin 38 g/L.

630 A 62-year-old woman presents to her GP with increasing tiredness, thirst, polyuria and recurrent epigastric pain. Normal full blood count, glucose and ESR. Urea 10.9 mmol/L, creatinine 135 mmol/L, calcium 3.28 mmol/L, phosphate 0.69 mmol/L, alkaline phosphatase 172 IU/L and albumin 39 g/L.

Theme: Amenorrhoea

Options

- A. Thyrotoxicosis
- B. Hypothyroidism
- C. Prolactinoma
- D. Pregnancy
- E. Menopause
- F. Primary ovarian failure
- G. Hypogonadal hypogonadism
- H. Polycystic ovary syndrome
- I. Cryptomenorrhoea
- J. Turner's syndrome
- K. Bulimia nervosa
- L. Anorexia nervosa

Instructions

For each case, choose the single most appropriate diagnosis from the list of options above. Each option may be used once, more than once or not at all.

631 A 17-year-old woman presents with a 3-month history of secondary amenorrhoea. She admits to binge eating and is concerned about being overweight. She goes to the gym daily and her BMI is 17.

632 A 37-year-old woman presents with a 4-month history of secondary amenorrhoea, palpitations and weight loss of 5 kg despite a good appetite. Pregnancy test is negative.

633 An 18-year-old woman presents with a 6-month history of secondary amenorrhoea, hirsutism and weight gain of 4 kg. She has suffered from irregular periods since menarche at the age of 13. Her BMI is 31.

634 A 17-year-old virgin with normal secondary sexual characteristics presents to her GP with primary amenorrhoea. O/E: a bluish bulge is seen just inside the hymen and the uterus shows 12 weeks' gestation.

635 A 42-year-old woman presents with a 4-month history of secondary amenorrhoea, recurrent headaches and reduced visual acuity. On further questioning, she admits to occasional staining of her bra with breast secretion.

Theme: Abdominal pain

Options

A. Perforated duodenal ulcer
B. Perforated diverticular disease
C. Gastritis
D. Small bowel obstruction
E. Large bowel obstruction
F. Diverticulitis
G. Gastric ulcer
H. Duodenal ulcer
I. Acute septic peritonitis
J. Acute appendicitis
K. Ischaemic colitis
L. Ulcerative colitis

Instructions

For each case, choose the single most appropriate diagnosis from the list of options above. Each option may be used once, more than once or not at all.

636 An 81-year-old woman presents with a 4-day history of recurrent lower abdominal pain, distension and absolute constipation. O/E: distended abdomen which is soft and non-tender on palpation. Percussion is hyperresonant.

637 A 52-year-old man presents with a 6-hour history of severe persistent epigastric pain. O/E: he appears very distressed, with pain, blood pressure is 110/60 mmHg, pulse is 120 bpm, his abdomen is very tender particularly at the epigastrium, with guarding rigidity. Bowel sounds are absent.

638 A 47-year-old man presents with a 4-day history of worsening periumbilical colicky pain, vomiting and abdominal distension. He last opened his bowels 2 days ago. His past medical history is unremarkable apart from a hernia surgery which was performed 2 years ago.

639 A 79-year-old woman with a long history of constipation presents with a 5-day history of worsening left iliac fossa pain and feeling generally unwell. O/E: temperature is 37.6°C, tender left iliac fossa with guarding rigidity.

640 A 78-year-old heavy smoker with a history of diabetes mellitus, hypertension and ischaemic heart disease presents with a 5-day history of left iliac fossa pain and bloody diarrhoea. Stool cultures are negative. Colonoscopy shows an ulcer at the rectum.

Theme: Rectal bleeding

Options
- A. Ulcerative colitis
- B. Crohn's disease
- C. Infectious colitis
- D. Ischaemic colitis
- E. Anal fissure
- F. Haemorrhoids
- G. Bleeding disorder
- H. Clotting disorder
- I. Diverticular disease
- J. Anal carcinoma
- K. Colonic carcinoma
- L. Colonic polyp

Instructions

For each case, choose the single most appropriate diagnosis from the list of options above. Each option may be used once, more than once or not at all.

641 A 24-year-old man presents with a 10-day history of bloody diarrhoea and abdominal cramp-like pain. Flexible sigmoidoscopy shows diffuse mucosal erythema. Biopsy shows oedema and inflammatory changes. Stool culture grows *E. coli*.

642 A 23-year-old woman presents with a 4-month history of bloody diarrhoea, abdominal pain and weight loss of 7 kg. O/E: swollen lips, buccal ulcers and raised red tender lesions on the shins. Colonoscopy shows multiple rectal ulcers with a normal mucosa in between.

643 A 30-year-old woman presents with a 3-month history of bloody diarrhoea and colicky abdominal pain. Colonoscopy shows diffuse mucosal erythema throughout the rectum and descending colon. Stool cultures are negative.

644 A 72-year-old man presents with a 2-month history of intermittent rectal bleeding, constipation and weight loss of 5 kg. Plain abdominal X-ray and proctoscopy are normal. Full blood count shows microcytic anaemia.

645 A 33-year-old man presents with a 2-month history of occasional painless bright rectal bleeding lining the stools and also on tissue paper. Full blood count is normal.

Theme: Eye drops

Options
- A. Timolol
- B. Pilocarpine
- C. Azelastine
- D. Guanethidine
- E. Tropicamide
- F. Phenylephrine
- G. Atropine
- H. Fluorescein
- I. Carbachol
- J. Hypromellose
- K. Dipivefrine
- L. Apraclonidine

Instructions

For each case, choose the single most appropriate eye drops from the list of options above. Each option may be used once, more than once or not at all.

646 A 68-year-old type 2 diabetic man arrives for his annual follow-up at the diabetes clinic. A mydriatic is needed for fundoscopy.

647 A 21-year-old man is referred to the ophthalmology clinic with a 4-year history of congested eyes and lacrimation occurring every spring, lasting for about 2 months.

648 A 71-year-old man under treatment for non-Hodgkin's lymphoma presents with a 2-day history of severe left ocular pain and photophobia. O/E: the left eye is very congested and multiple small vesicles are noted at the nose.

649 A fit and healthy 69-year-old woman visits her optician to change her reading glasses. Fundoscopy shows cupping of the optic disc.

650 A 49-year-old woman is referred to the rheumatology clinic with a 4-month history of itchy eyes, dry mouth and bilateral parotid enlargement. Schirmer's test is positive.

Theme: Urinary symptoms in children

Options

- A. Henoch–Schönlein purpura
- B. Bacterial cystitis
- C. Renal vein thrombosis
- D. Acute pyelonephritis
- E. Vesicoureteric reflux
- F. Haemolytic uraemic syndrome
- G. Nephroblastoma
- H. Acute glomerulonephritis
- I. Congenital polycystic kidneys
- J. Benign recurrent haematuria
- K. Horseshoe kidney
- L. Renal TB

Instructions

For each case, choose the single most appropriate diagnosis from the list of options above. Each option may be used once, more than once or not at all.

651 A 4-year-old girl presents with dysuria, frequency of micturition and itching in the pubic region.

652 A 5-year-old girl presents with oliguria, haematuria and diffuse oedema. She had a sore throat 3 weeks earlier.

653 A 7-year-old boy with a history of recurrent painless haematuria is fully investigated and all his results are normal (including IVU and abdominal ultrasound scan).

654 A 2-year-old girl presents with fever and marked abdominal distension. Urinalysis shows microscopic haematuria. There is no family history of any renal disease.

655 A 12-year-old boy presents with acute abdominal pain. He has a 3-month history of bilateral knee pain. O/E: skin rash mainly in his lower limbs, urinalysis shows microscopic haematuria.

Theme: Viral infections in children

Options

A. Rotavirus
B. Hepatitis B virus
C. *Molluscum contagiosum*
D. Cytomegalovirus
E. Epstein–Barr virus
F. Rubella virus
G. Mumps virus
H. Influenza virus
I. Parainfluenza virus
J. Poliomyelitis virus
K. Coxsackie virus
L. Measles virus

Instructions

For each case, choose the single most appropriate viral infection from the list of options above. Each option may be used once, more than once or not at all.

656 A 4-year-old child develops papular lesions with umbilicated centres on his trunk. They disappear within 7 months. The child remains well throughout.

657 A 6-month-old baby presents with fever, cough and tachypnoea. Chest X-ray shows bilateral widespread shadows. His mother is HIV positive.

658 The 2-year-old son of Albanian refugees presents with fever, increased salivation and a swollen left cheek.

659 A 2-year-old boy presents with a 12-hour history of fever, cough and hoarseness of voice. While waiting in A&E, he develops stridor.

660 A 5-year-old child develops severe diarrhoea, nausea and vomiting 1 day after returning from a school trip.

Theme: Haematemesis

Options

A. Erosive gastritis
B. Oesophageal carcinoma
C. Oesophageal varices
D. Peptic ulcer
E. Mallory–Weiss tear
F. Gastric leiomyoma
G. Hiatus hernia
H. Oesophagitis
I. Gastric carcinoma
J. Zollinger–Ellison syndrome
K. Bleeding disorder
L. Clotting disorder

Instructions

For each case, choose the single most appropriate diagnosis from the list of options above. Each option may be used once, more than once or not at all.

661 A 25-year-old painter presents early on a Sunday morning with vomiting of fresh blood. He admits to drinking 9 pints of beer on Saturday night. He had vomited several times before finally vomiting about 40 cc of fresh blood.

662 A 76-year-old woman is admitted to ITU with extensive burns and hypotension. She is resuscitated but within 24 hours she vomits 200 cc of coffee-ground fluid.

663 A 69-year-old heavy smoker presents with recurrent coffee-ground vomiting and weight loss of 14 kg over the last 3 months. He also admits to loss of appetite, epigastric discomfort and sensation of fullness after small meals.

664 A 54-year-old Egyptian farmer with a history of schistosomiasis presents with haematemesis and melaena. O/E: palpable hepatosplenomegaly and caput medusae.

665 A 42-year-old woman with a history of recurrent peptic ulcers, which didn't respond in the past to ranitidine, presents with coffee-ground vomiting. Endoscopy shows multiple duodenal ulcers. Abdominal CT scan shows a small pancreatic mass.

Theme: Methods of contraception

Options

- A. Periodic abstinence
- B. Condom
- C. Intrauterine contraceptive device
- D. Combined oral contraceptive pill
- E. Coitus interruptus
- F. Sterilisation
- G. Vaginal diaphragm
- H. Cervical cap
- I. Depot progesterone
- J. Progesterone-only contraceptive pill
- K. Spermicide
- L. Mifepristone

Instructions

For each statement, choose the single most appropriate method of contraception from the list of options above. Each option may be used once, more than once or not at all.

666 Is contraindicated in migraine or a history of deep venous thrombosis. *D*

667 Is contraindicated if either partner is not sure whether they would like to have children in the future. *F*

668 Is only suitable in a stable relationship. *A*

669 Is absolutely contraindicated if there is a previous history of ectopic pregnancy or uterine abnormality. *C*

670 Is unreliable if the menstrual cycles are irregular. *A*

671 Is probably the least reliable method of contraception. *E*

672 Reduces the risk of ovarian and endometrial carcinoma. *D*

673 Improves primary dysmenorrhoea. *D*

Theme: Pupillary abnormalities

Options

A. Marcus Gunn pupil
B. Horner's syndrome
C. Third cranial nerve palsy
D. Iritis
E. Iridectomy
F. Opiate toxicity
G. Aphakia
H. Argyll Robertson pupil
I. Holmes–Adie pupil
J. Glaucoma
K. Medullary lesion
L. Brainstem death

Instructions

For each statement, choose the single most appropriate diagnosis from the list of options above. Each option may be used once, more than once or not at all.

674 The right pupil is slightly dilated, with absent direct papillary reflex but normal consensual light reflex. The left pupil is normal.

675 The left pupil is slightly dilated, with diminished direct and consensual papillary reflexes. The right pupil is normal. The knee jerk is absent.

676 The right pupil is small, with partial ptosis and slight enophthalmos. The left pupil is normal.

677 Both pupils are small and irregular. Accommodation reflex is present but light reflex is absent.

678 Bilateral, fixed and pinpoint pupils.

679 The left pupil is dilated and unreactive, with complete ptosis and lateral deviation of the eye.

Theme: Monitoring of medications

Options

    A. Thyroid function test
    B. Full blood count
    C. Serum creatinine phosphokinase
    D. INR
    E. aPTT
    F. Serum amylase
    G. Liver function test
    H. HbA1c
    I. ECG
    J. Drug serum levels
    K. Arterial blood gas
    L. Serum ferritin
    M. Urea and electrolytes

Instructions

For each medication, choose the single most appropriate investigation from the list of options above. Each option may be used once, more than once or not at all.

680 Digoxin
681 Ramipril
682 Fluconazole
683 Amiodarone
684 Insulin
685 Warfarin
686 Carbimazole
687 Heparin

Theme: Hoarseness of voice

Options

A. Acute bacterial laryngitis
B. Acute viral laryngitis
C. Chronic laryngitis
D. Laryngeal candidiasis
E. Tuberculous laryngitis
F. Myxoedema
G. Laryngeal papilloma
H. Laryngeal carcinoma
I. Sjögren's syndrome
J. Ortner's syndrome
K. Vocal cord nodules
L. Bronchial carcinoma

Instructions

For each case, choose the single most appropriate diagnosis from the list of options above. Each option may be used once, more than once or not at all.

688 A 69-year-old heavy smoker presents with a 7-week history of hoarseness of voice and weight loss. On laryngoscopy, the left vocal cord is near the midline and doesn't move. The larynx otherwise looks normal.

689 A 72-year-old heavy smoker with a long history of COPD presents with a 3-week history of hoarseness of voice. He has been on three different inhalers for at least 2 years. O/E: the throat is red with a few white patches. Laryngoscopy shows reddish larynx and vocal cords which move normally.

690 A 40-year-old auctioneer presents with a 6-week history of hoarseness of voice. He neither smokes nor drinks any alcohol. Laryngoscopy shows slightly reddish vocal cords with a small swelling at the junction of the anterior third and the posterior two-thirds of each vocal cord.

691 A 64-year-old heavy smoker and alcoholic presents with a 5-week history of hoarseness of voice. Laryngoscopy shows a greyish white swelling at the anterior third of the left vocal cord.

692 A fit and healthy 10-year-old boy presents with a 2-week history of hoarseness of voice. Laryngoscopy shows a pedunculated swelling on the left vocal cord.

693 A 42-year-old woman with a long history of mitral stenosis presents with progressive hoarseness of voice over the last few months. Chest X-ray shows a remarkably enlarged left atrium. Laryngoscopy shows normal larynx but the left vocal cord is near the midline and doesn't move.

Theme: Milestones in children

Options

- A. 0–2 months
- B. 2–5 months
- C. 4–7 months
- D. 7–10 months
- E. 11–14 months
- F. 14–18 months
- G. 18–24 months
- H. 3 years
- I. 4 years
- J. 5 years
- K. 6–8 years
- L. 8–10 years

Instructions

For each statement, choose the single most appropriate age from the list of options above. Each option may be used once, more than once or not at all.

694 Retains head in an upright position

695 Crawls

696 Talks in simple phrases

697 Develops concepts of size, shape, colour, place and time

698 Builds a tower of two blocks

699 Drinks from a cup

700 Tells a story

701 Rolls from back to front or to side

702 Dresses and undresses almost independently

703 Rides a bicycle

Theme: Prescribing medication in pregnancy

Options

A. Should be avoided as it may affect foetal blood pressure control and renal function.
B. Is not teratogenic.
C. May cause neonatal grey syndrome.
D. Should be avoided as it may cause virilisation of a female foetus.
E. May cause neonatal jaundice and methaemoglobinaemia.
F. Should be avoided as it may cause cardiac abnormalities.
G. May cause closure of foetal ductus arteriosus and persistent pulmonary hypertension in the newborn.
H. May cause abruptio placentae.
I. Is a recognised cause of ectopic pregnancy.
J. The dose must be halved in the second trimester of pregnancy.
K. May only be used in the first trimester of pregnancy.
L. Should be avoided as it increases the uterine tone.

Instructions

For each medication, choose the single most appropriate statement from the list of options above. Each option may be used once, more than once or not at all.

704 Ramipril
705 Danazol
706 Lithium
707 Misoprostol
708 Aspirin
709 Cephalexin
710 Dapsone
711 Chloramphenicol

Theme: Visual problems

Options

- A. Bitemporal hemianopia
- B. Third cranial nerve palsy
- C. Fourth cranial nerve palsy
- D. Sixth cranial nerve palsy
- E. Cortical blindness
- F. Cataract
- G. Background diabetic retinopathy
- H. Proliferative diabetic retinopathy
- I. Glaucoma
- J. Amaurosis fugax
- K. Optic atrophy
- L. Retrobulbar neuritis

Instructions

For each case, choose the single most appropriate diagnosis from the list of options above. Each option may be used once, more than once or not at all.

712 A 70-year-old heavy smoker with a long history of poorly controlled hypertension presents with a 2-hour history of sudden-onset blindness. Both eyes look normal. Fundoscopy is also normal.

713 A 44-year-old man presents to his GP with recurrent headaches and sweating. He noted that his shoes, gloves and ring no longer fit him. He also noted that he tends to bump into people while walking.

714 A 67-year-old woman presents to A&E with a 2-hour history of blindness in the right eye which felt like a curtain descending over her vision. Within half an hour, her vision returns to normal. General examination, fundoscopy, chest X-ray and routine blood tests are all normal.

715 A 34-year-old nurse presents with a 3-month history of intermittent numbness and tingling in her left arm and blurring of vision. Visual field studies confirm loss of central vision in the left eye. Fundoscopy is normal.

716 A 56-year-old alcoholic with no fixed abode presents with a 3-month history of reduced visual acuity. Fundoscopy shows pale discs but the retina seems normal.

Theme: Muscle weakness

Options

    A. Hypocalcaemia
    B. Hypokalaemia
    C. Spinal cord compression
    D. Left anterior cerebral artery infarct
    E. Left middle cerebral artery infarct
    F. Multiple sclerosis
    G. Guillain–Barré syndrome
    H. Myasthenia gravis
    I. Motor neurone disease
    J. Poliomyelitis
    K. Cerebellar syndrome
    L. Alcoholic myopathy
    M. Right middle cerebral artery infarct
    N. Right anterior cerebral artery infarct

Instructions

For each case, choose the single most appropriate diagnosis from the list of options above. Each option may be used once, more than once or not at all.

717 A 27-year-old woman with a history of vitiligo and autoimmune thyroid disease presents with a 2-week history of worsening fatiguability and diplopia. Tensilon test is positive.

718 A 79-year-old hypertensive woman presents with sudden weakness of the right side of her body, expressive dysphasia and right-side sensory inattention.

719 A 64-year-old man with metastatic prostatic carcinoma presents with a 1-week history of worsening lower limb weakness, constipation and recurrent falls. O/E: bilateral weakness of both lower limbs (grade 4/5), hyperreflexia, extensor plantars and a sensory level at T9.

720 A 39-year-old woman presents with a 1-week history of lower limb weakness following acute gastroenteritis. O/E: bilateral distal weakness of both lower limbs (grade 4/5), diminished reflexes and absent plantars. Superficial sensation is also reduced. The rest of neurological examination is unremarkable.

721 A 56-year-old man presents with a 4-month history of pain and weakness of all limbs. O/E: clubbing, spider naevi, Dupuytren's contracture and proximal myopathy.

722 A 62-year-old woman presents with progressive asymmetrical weakness of all limbs, dysphagia and nasal regurgitation. O/E: wasting and fasciculation of all limbs, tongue is flaccid and fasciculating and the jaw jerk is absent. There is no sensory loss. Ocular movement and cerebellar function are intact.

Theme: Physical signs in ophthalmology

Options

A. Tunnel vision
B. Bitemporal hemianopia
C. Cherry red spot
D. Argyll Robertson pupil
E. Holmes–Adie pupil
F. Angioid streaks
G. Flame-shaped haemorrhages
H. Homonymous hemianopia
I. Hard exudates
J. Cotton wool patches
K. Heterochromia of the iris (heterochromia iridum)
L. Exophthalmos

Instructions

For each diagnosis, choose the single most appropriate physical sign from the list of options above. Each option may be used once, more than once or not at all.

723 Retinitis pigmentosa
724 Neurosyphilis
725 Central retinal artery occlusion
726 Pituitary tumour (macroadenoma)
727 Cerebrovascular accident
728 Fuchs' heterochromic iridocyclitis
729 Pseudoxanthoma elasticum
730 Graves' disease

Theme: Dysphagia

Options

- A. Oesophageal candidiasis
- B. Pharyngeal pouch (Zenker's diverticulum)
- C. Scleroderma
- D. Chagas' disease
- E. Pharyngeal web
- F. Myasthenia gravis
- G. Bulbar palsy
- H. Pseudobulbar palsy
- I. Gastro-oesophageal reflux disease (GORD)
- J. Herpetic oesophagitis
- K. Cardiac achalasia
- L. Oesophageal carcinoma

Instructions

For each case, choose the single most appropriate diagnosis from the list of options above. Each option may be used once, more than once or not at all.

731 A 50-year-old man presents with a 4-month history of progressive dysphagia, nasal regurgitation and dysarthria. O/E: the tongue is flaccid and fasciculating, palatal movement and jaw jerk are both absent. Ocular movement is normal.

732 A 62-year-old man presents with a 4-month history of progressive dysphagia, mainly to solids, and weight loss of 3 kg. Investigations show iron deficiency anaemia and hypoalbuminaemia.

733 A 42-year-old obese woman presents with a 9-month history of burning epigastric pain which is worse at night or after oily food. Over the last 2 weeks she has developed occasional dysphagia to solids. Endoscopy shows hiatus hernia, inflammation and stricture at the lower third of the oesophagus.

734 A 35-year-old woman presents with a 2-month history of chest pain, dysphagia and regurgitation of solids and fluids. Barium swallow shows beak-like tapering of the lower third of the oesophagus.

735 A 31-year-old HIV-positive man presents with a 1-week history of dysphagia and odynophagia, mainly to solids. Barium swallow shows multiple oesophageal ulcers.

Theme: Psychiatric illness

Options

A. Post-traumatic stress disorder
B. Bereavement reaction
C. Generalised anxiety disorder
D. Agoraphobia
E. Dementia
F. Paranoid schizophrenia
G. Panic disorder
H. Bipolar disorder
I. Depression
J. Mania
K. Chronic fatigue syndrome
L. Delirium

Instructions

For each case, choose the single most appropriate diagnosis from the list of options above. Each option may be used once, more than once or not at all.

736 A 27-year-old man presents with palpitations, shortness of breath and low mood. He feels 'uncomfortable', particularly when he goes shopping. He recently lost his job as a musician and he has been finding it increasingly difficult to perform in the presence of an audience.

737 A 53-year-old woman who lost her husband in an accident 5 months ago presents with poor memory and concentration. She is also complaining of insomnia and unexplained anger.

738 A 26-year-old man reports hearing voices swearing at him. He claims to be closely followed by the CIA through satellites. One year ago he lost his job as a computer programmer due to his poor concentration and bizarre behaviour.

739 A 42-year-old woman presents with tiredness with minimal effort, with rest bringing little relief. She complains of lack of energy, headache, poor memory and muscle ache. Physical examination and investigations are normal.

740 A 70-year-old inpatient at a surgical ward becomes increasingly confused over 12 hours. He is agitated, completely disorientated and very sweaty.

Theme: ECG findings in arrhythmias and conduction defects

Options

A. Normal P waves and PR interval. Wide QRS complexes with deep S waves in lead V_6.

B. Abnormal P waves. Normal QRS complexes. Ventricular rate is regular at 180 bpm.

C. Absent P waves. Normal QRS complexes. Ventricular rate is irregular at 135 bpm.

D. Saw-tooth baseline. Normal QRS complexes. Ventricular rate is regular at 150 bpm.

E. Normal P waves. Normal QRS complexes. Ventricular rate is regular at 140 bpm.

F. Absent P waves. Predominantly negative QRS complexes in leads V_4 to V_6.

G. Short PR interval. Delta waves. Ventricular rate is regular at 90 bpm.

H. A bizarre and broadened QRS complex followed by a T wave pointing in the opposite direction to the QRS component. The QRS is not preceded by a P wave.

I. Normal and regular P waves and QRS complexes. Constantly prolonged PR interval. Ventricular rate is 70 bpm.

J. Normal and regular P waves and QRS complexes. Progressive lengthening of PR interval followed by one non-conducted beat. Ventricular rate is 74 bpm.

K. P wave rate is 86 per minute. QRS wave rate is 35 per minute. No relationship between P waves and QRS complexes.

L. Normal P waves and PR interval. Wide QRS complexes with inverted T waves in the lateral leads.

Instructions

For each arrhythmia, choose the single most appropriate ECG description from the list of options above. Each option may be used once, more than once or not at all.

741 Ventricular tachycardia

742 Ventricular extrasystole

743 Atrial flutter

744 Wolff–Parkinson–White syndrome

745 Atrial tachycardia

746 Atrial fibrillation

747 First-degree heart block

748 Sinus tachycardia

Theme: Interpretation of blood results

Options

A. Old age
B. Anaemia of chronic disease
C. Iron deficiency anaemia
D. Myelodysplasia
E. Folate deficiency anaemia
F. Chronic myeloid leukaemia
G. Alcoholic liver disease
H. Chronic lymphocytic leukaemia
I. β-thalassaemia minor
J. β-thalassaemia major
K. Cytotoxic drugs
L. Vitamin B$_{12}$ deficiency

Instructions

For each case, choose the single most appropriate diagnosis from the list of options above. Each option may be used once, more than once or not at all.

749 A 59-year-old man: Hb 13.1 g/dL, MCV 105 fL, WCC 6.1 × 10^9/L and platelets 118 × 10^9/L. Blood film shows target cells and hypersegmented neutrophils.

750 A 22-year-old man undergoes routine investigations for medical insurance: Hb 12.1 g/dL, MCV 73 fL, MCH 27 g/dL, RBC count 6.5 × 10^{12}/L, WCC 7.2 × 10^9/L, platelets 290 × 10^9/L and ferritin 200 µg/L.

751 A 78-year-old woman is investigated for tiredness and lethargy: Hb 9.3 g/dL, MCV 103 fL, WCC 3.8 × 10^9/L (lymphocytes 1.4, neutrophils 1.2, monocytes 0.9 and myeloblasts 0.1) and platelets 125 × 10^9/L.

752 A 77-year-old diabetic and hypertensive woman attends for her routine check up: Hb 11.4 g/dL, MCV 81 fL, WCC 8.0 × 10^9/L, platelets 440 × 10^9/L and ferritin 320 µg/L, serum iron 42 µg/dL, TIBC 174 µg/dL.

753 A 63-year-old man with a long history of epilepsy: Hb 10 g/dL, MCV 111 fL, WCC 3.8 × 10^9/L (lymphocytes 2.3 and neutrophils 1.2) and platelets 230 × 10^9/L.

754 A 70-year-old asymptomatic man: Hb 10.6 g/dL, MCV 86 fL, MCH 31 g/dL, WCC 19 × 10^9/L, platelets 185 × 10^9/L and direct antiglobulin test is positive.

Theme: Arthritis

Options

- A. Osteoarthritis
- B. Haemarthrosis
- C. Onchronosis
- D. Gout
- E. Pseudogout
- F. Septic arthritis
- G. Charcot joint
- H. Tuberculous arthritis
- I. Ankylosing spondylitis
- J. Rheumatoid arthritis
- K. Systemic lupus erythematosus
- L. Reiter's syndrome

Instructions

For each case, choose the single most appropriate diagnosis from the list of options above. Each option may be used once, more than once or not at all.

755 A 32-year-old man presents to A&E with a red, hot, tender and swollen left knee. He injured his left knee in a football game 2 days earlier and 20 mL of blood had then been aspirated in A&E.

756 A 62-year-old obese and hypertensive man who was recently started on a diuretic presents with a painful right toe. O/E: red, hot, swollen and tender interphalangeal joint of the right big toe.

757 A 70-year-old man with a 40-year history of diabetes mellitus noted progressive painless swelling of his right ankle over the last few months. O/E: loss of superficial and deep sensation distal to the right knee. X-ray of the right ankle shows gross deformity.

758 A 64-year-old man with a history of haemochromatosis presents with a 2-month history of bilateral knee pain. X-ray of knees shows a rim of intraarticular calcification. Serum calcium and urate are normal.

759 A 32-year-old man presents with a 2-week history of arthritis, dysuria and dry gritty eyes. He suffered from gastroenteritis 4 weeks ago.

Theme: Vitamin deficiency

Options

    A. Vitamin A deficiency
    B. Vitamin B_3 (niacin) deficiency
    C. Vitamin C deficiency
    D. Vitamin D deficiency
    E. Vitamin E deficiency
    F. Folate deficiency
    G. Vitamin B_1 (thiamine) deficiency
    H. Vitamin B_2 (riboflavin) deficiency
    I. Vitamin B_6 (pyridoxine) deficiency
    J. Vitamin B_{12} (cobalamin) deficiency
    K. Vitamin K deficiency

Instructions

For each description, choose the single most appropriate diagnosis from the list of options above. Each option may be used once, more than once or not at all.

760 Bowing of the legs, lumbar lordosis and pigeon chest.

761 Bruising, epistaxis, haemoptysis, haematuria, haematemesis and melaena.

762 Peripheral neuropathy, loss of short-term memory, ankle oedema, ataxia, nystagmus and confabulation.

763 Gingivitis, bleeding gums, bruises, papular rash and petechial haemorrhages.

764 Sore throat, swollen mucous membranes, oral ulcers, anaemia and dermatitis.

765 Dermatitis, diarrhoea and dementia.

766 Anaemia, memory loss, optic neuritis, impaired peripheral sensation and abnormal gait.

Theme: Bleeding in pregnancy

Options

- A. Cervical carcinoma
- B. Cervical erosion
- C. Velamentous insertion of the cord
- D. Ectopic pregnancy
- E. Placenta praevia
- F. Hydatidiform (vesicular) mole
- G. Choriocarcinoma
- H. Abruptio placenta
- I. Withdrawal bleeding
- J. Bleeding disorder
- K. Clotting disorder
- L. Endometrial carcinoma

Instructions

For each case, choose the single most appropriate diagnosis from the list of options above. Each option may be used once, more than once or not at all.

767 A 34-year-old para 4+2 presents with painless dark brown bleeding of about 5 cc in volume. She had had intercourse 1 day earlier.

768 A 24-year-old woman is brought to A&E after collapsing at work. Her last period was 8 weeks ago. She is complaining of severe lower abdominal pain.

769 A 32-year-old Chinese woman who is 19 weeks pregnant presents with severe nausea, vomiting and heavy vaginal bleeding. O/E: uterus is large for date.

770 A 37-year-old para 3+1 who is 34 weeks pregnant presents with painless fresh vaginal bleeding of about 150 cc in volume.

771 A 29-year-old primigravida is in labour. Twenty minutes after rupture of membranes, the foetal heart rate drops suddenly. Her vital signs all remain normal.

Theme: Mode of inheritance

Options

- A. Haemophilia A
- B. Turner's syndrome
- C. Familial hypophosphataemic rickets
- D. Rett syndrome
- E. Marfan's syndrome
- F. Leber's optic atrophy
- G. Myotonic dystrophy
- H. Cystic fibrosis
- I. Hypertrichosis pinnae (hairy ear pinna)
- J. Angina pectoris
- K. Osteoarthritis
- L. Gout

Instructions

For each mode of inheritance, choose the single most appropriate condition from the list of options above. Each option may be used once, more than once or not at all.

772 Autosomal dominant

773 Autosomal recessive

774 X-linked dominant

775 X-linked recessive

776 Y-linked

777 Mitochondrial DNA-related inheritance

778 Autosomal dominant with genetic anticipation

Theme: Management of labour

Options

A. CTG monitoring
B. Ultrasound scan
C. Oxygen
D. Oxytocin
E. Intravenous fluids
F. Foetal blood sampling
G. Forceps
H. Emergency Caesarean section
I. Elective Caesarean section
J. Blood transfusion
K. Diamorphine
L. Regular observation

Instructions

For each case, choose the single most appropriate management step from the list of options above. Each option may be used once, more than once or not at all.

779 A 31-year-old primiparous woman is fully dilated for 4 hours and has been pushing for 1.5 hours. The foetal head is in occipito-posterior position 4 cm below the ischial spine.

780 A 27-year-old primiparous woman is admitted to hospital 1 hour after rupture of her membranes. She is 39 weeks pregnant but the baby is known to be small for date.

781 A 34-year-old obese multiparous woman presents in early labour. O/E: the presenting part has not engaged to the pelvic outlet.

782 A 32-year-old multiparous woman is fully dilated for 1 hour and the CTG shows variable decelerations.

783 A 29-year-old primiparous woman is admitted 2 hours after start of labour at 39 weeks' gestation. O/E: the cervix is 3 cm dilated and meconium is seen. CTG shows evidence of foetal distress.

Theme: Classification of medication in psychotherapy

Options

A. Tricyclic antidepressant (TCA)
B. Serotonin–norepinephrine reuptake inhibitor (SNRI)
C. Selective serotonin reuptake inhibitor (SSRI)
D. Monoamine oxidase inhibitor (MAOI)
E. Reversible inhibitor of monoamine oxidase A (RIMA)
F. Mood stabiliser
G. Typical antipsychotic
H. Atypical antipsychotic
I. Benzodiazepine
J. Analgesic
K. Hypnotic

Instructions

For each medication, choose the single most appropriate class from the list of options above. Each option may be used once, more than once or not at all.

784 Fluoxetine
785 Phenelzine
786 Lithium
787 Amitriptyline
788 Diazepam
789 Venlafaxine
790 Chlorpromazine
791 Moclobemide
792 Risperidone

Theme: Neonatal jaundice

Options

- A. Galactosaemia
- B. Glucose-6-phosphate dehydrogenase (G6PD) deficiency
- C. Crigler–Najjar syndrome
- D. Gilbert's syndrome
- E. Hepatitis C
- F. Congenital toxoplasmosis
- G. Biliary atresia
- H. Breast milk jaundice
- I. Rhesus incompatibility
- J. ABO incompatibility
- K. Budd–Chiari syndrome
- L. Physiological jaundice

Instructions

For each case, choose the single most appropriate diagnosis from the list of options above. Each option may be used once, more than once or not at all.

793 A full-term newborn becomes jaundiced 14 hours after delivery. His blood results confirm indirect bilirubinaemia and metabolic acidosis. His parents are both rhesus negative.

794 A full-term newborn develops jaundice at day three, which peaks at day seven, then fully recovers by day 14. His blood results showed indirect bilirubinaemia with normal liver function tests (while he was jaundiced).

795 A full-term newborn develops jaundice at day four, which gradually worsens over the next 2 weeks. His blood results showed direct bilirubinaemia.

796 A preterm newborn is jaundiced at birth. O/E: hepatosplenomegaly and congested eyes. Full blood count shows thrombocytopenia.

797 A healthy full-term newborn becomes jaundiced at day two. His total bilirubin is 10 mg/dL. His jaundice gradually disappears over the next few days.

Theme: Physical signs in dermatology

Options

- A. Exclamation-mark hair
- B. Perifollicular haemorrhage
- C. Spider naevi
- D. De Morgan's spots
- E. Wheal
- F. Café au lait spots
- G. Nail fold infarcts
- H. Yellow nails
- I. Calcinosis
- J. Onycholysis
- K. Erythema multiforme
- L. Erythema nodosum

Instructions

For each diagnosis, choose the single most appropriate physical sign from the list of options above. Each option may be used once, more than once or not at all.

798 Urticaria
799 Psoriasis
800 Scurvy
801 Alcoholic liver disease
802 Alopecia areata
803 Tuberous sclerosis
804 Ulcerative colitis
805 Normal feature in Caucasians

Theme: Neck swellings

Options

- A. Multinodular goitre
- B. Sternomastoid tumour
- C. Lymphoma
- D. Thyroglossal cyst
- E. Sebaceous cyst
- F. Cystic hygroma
- G. Cervical rib
- H. Pharyngeal pouch (Zenker's diverticulum)
- I. Tonsillitis
- J. Branchial cleft cyst
- K. Metastatic carcinoma
- L. Teratoma

Instructions

For each case, choose the single most appropriate diagnosis from the list of options above. Each option may be used once, more than once or not at all.

806 A 15-year-old girl presents with a painless swelling in the upper part of the right side of the neck. O/E: 5-cm rounded, smooth, non-tender and fluctuant swelling is felt beneath the upper third of the sternomastoid.

807 A 71-year-old man presents with a painless, slowly growing swelling in the posterior triangle of the neck. He has been complaining of night fever, night sweats and weight loss for about 3 months. O/E: axillary lymph nodes are palpable.

808 A 68-year-old heavy smoker presents with a painless, slowly growing swelling in the anterior triangle of the neck. He notes that his voice has been hoarse for at least 3 months. O/E: 2-cm rounded, hard, non-tender swelling deep to the sternomastoid muscle.

809 A 77-year-old man presents with dysphagia, regurgitation of food and chronic cough. O/E: 6-cm soft, smooth, non-tender and compressible swelling behind the sternomastoid and inferior to the thyroid cartilage, on the left side of the neck.

810 A 17-year-old man presents with a painless swelling in the midline of the neck, just in front of the trachea. The swelling moves on swallowing and protrusion of the tongue.

Theme: Prescribing antimicrobials

Options

- A. Trimethoprim
- B. Piperacillin and tobramycin
- C. Azithromycin
- D. Augmentin and clarithromycin
- E. Benzyl penicillin and flucloxacillin
- F. Acyclovir
- G. Metronidazole
- H. Flucloxacillin and fusidic acid
- I. Fluconazole
- J. Isoniazid, rifampicin, ethambutol and pyrazinamide
- K. Clotrimazole
- L. Pyrazinamide

Instructions

For each infection, choose the single most appropriate antibiotic(s) from the list of options above. Each option may be used once, more than once or not at all.

811 Pulmonary tuberculosis

812 Cellulitis

813 Pseudomembranous colitis

814 Hospital-acquired pneumonia

815 Urinary tract infection

816 Community-acquired pneumonia

817 Staphylococcal osteomyelitis

818 *Chlamydia trachomatis*

Theme: Chromosomal abnormalities

Options

A. Edwards' syndrome
B. Turner's syndrome
C. Down's syndrome
D. Klinefelter's syndrome
E. Patau's syndrome
F. Prader–Willi syndrome
G. Cri-du-chat syndrome
H. Double Y syndrome
I. Fragile X syndrome
J. Triple X syndrome

Instructions

For each case, choose the single most appropriate diagnosis from the list of options above. Each option may be used once, more than once or not at all.

819 A male neonate with cleft lip and palate, low-set ears and polydactyly. Chromosome analysis confirms a genotype of 47XY.

820 A 17-year-old boy with low IQ, testicular atrophy, gynaecomastia and tall stature. Chromosome analysis confirms a genotype of 47XXY.

821 A male neonate with low-set ears, micrognathia, cleft lip and palate, occipital prominence, polydactyly and rocker-bottom feet. Chromosome analysis confirms a genotype of 47XY.

822 A 4-year-old boy with simian creases, epicanthal folds, slanting eyes, short stature and pansystolic murmur loudest over the left-fourth parasternal space.

823 A 16-year-old girl with primary amenorrhoea, webbing of the neck, low hairline, nail hypoplasia and wide-spaced nipples.

Theme: Menorrhagia

Options

A. Physiological
B. Intrauterine contraceptive device
C. Depression
D. Pelvic inflammatory disease
E. Adenomyosis
F. Hypothyroidism
G. Uterine fibroids
H. Cervical carcinoma
I. Chronic alcoholism
J. Endometrial carcinoma
K. Bleeding disorder
L. Clotting disorder

Instructions

For each case, choose the single most appropriate diagnosis from the list of options above. Each option may be used once, more than once or not at all.

824 A 26-year-old woman who has been treated twice for chlamydial urethritis over the last 2 years presents with dyspareunia, irregular heavy periods and lower abdominal discomfort. On examination her temperature is 37.3°C.

825 A 34-year-old woman presents with a 2-year history of gradually worsening painless menorrhagia. O/E: she is pale and has an enlarged bulky uterus.

826 A 28-year-old woman presents with a 2-month history of menorrhagia. She describes bleeding for 5 days every 29 days, which is of average amount. General and pelvic examination is normal. Full blood count, bleeding time, clotting profile and renal function tests are all normal.

827 A 38-year-old woman presents with a 6-month history of severe menorrhagia and lower abdominal pain. O/E: she is pale and has an enlarged tender uterus equivalent to a 14-week pregnancy. She is treated by a hysterectomy.

828 An obese 42-year-old woman presents with a 3-month history of menorrhagia and intermenstrual bleeding. General and pelvic examination is unremarkable. Full blood count shows mild anaemia. Clotting profile, liver function tests and ultrasound are normal. Diagnosis is confirmed by D&C.

Theme: Choice of contraception

Options

    A. Condom

    B. Vasectomy

    C. Intrauterine contraceptive device

    D. Depo-Provera (progesterone depot injection)

    E. Progesterone-only contraceptive pill

    F. Combined oral contraceptive pill

    G. Post-coital high-dose levonorgestrel

    H. Laparoscopic sterilisation

    I. Spermicide

    J. Mifepristone

    K. Norplant (progesterone implant)

Instructions

For each case, choose the single most appropriate contraception from the list of options above. Each option may be used once, more than once or not at all.

829 A 20-year-old waitress discovers that her partner is hepatitis C positive. She still wishes to continue her relationship with him.

830 A 28-year-old lawyer suffering from irregular, heavy and painful periods attends her GP surgery asking for contraception.

831 A 37-year-old housewife who has four children attends her GP surgery asking for contraception. She has completed her family. She is not keen on oral contraceptive pills or any surgical intervention and her husband refuses to have a vasectomy or use condoms. A pelvic ultrasound scan shows two large uterine fibroids.

832 A 23-year-old air hostess with a history of migraine attends her GP surgery asking for contraception for at least 1 year. Her partner refuses to use condoms.

833 A 20-year-old student had unprotected intercourse 2 days prior to attending her GP surgery. She is concerned that she might become pregnant.

834 A 38-year-old smoker with two children attends her GP surgery asking for contraception. Two years ago, she had had a left lumpectomy performed for breast cancer, which was complicated by a left femoral thrombosis. In view of her negative experience with her lumpectomy, she is not keen on any further surgical interventions. Her partner refuses to use condoms or have a vasectomy.

Theme: Haematuria

Options

- A. Ureteric stone
- B. Renal tuberculosis
- C. Renal stone
- D. Polycystic kidneys
- E. Haemophilia
- F. Cystitis
- G. Renal cell carcinoma
- H. Nephroblastoma
- I. Prostatic carcinoma
- J. Bladder carcinoma
- K. Acute pyelonephritis
- L. Acute glomerulonephritis

Instructions

For each case, choose the single most appropriate diagnosis from the list of options above. Each option may be used once, more than once or not at all.

835 A 14-year-old boy presents with a 2-month history of intermittent haematuria and right loin pain. O/E: temperature is 36.8°C, blood pressure is 180/105 mmHg and pulse is 90 bpm. Abdominal examination reveals bilateral ballottable masses in both loins. Marked plethora is also noted. The patient's father was started on haemodialysis at the age of 29 years.

836 A 54-year-old man presents with a 3-month history of recurrent right-side renal colic. MSU shows aseptic pyuria, while urinalysis shows microscopic haematuria. Plain abdominal X-ray is unremarkable. IVU shows an obstructed right pelvicalyceal system and a filling defect in the proximal right ureter.

837 A 72-year-old heavy smoker presents at A&E with painless frank haematuria. He is otherwise fit and well, but reports exposure to aniline dyes 49 years ago. General examination is unremarkable. Renal function and PSA are normal.

838 A 50-year-old man presents with a 2-month history of haematuria, left loin pain, night sweating and weight loss of 5 kg. O/E: there is a palpable mass in the left loin and also a left varicocele.

839 A 74-year-old man presents with frank haematuria. He noticed that blood came at the beginning of the stream. He also has a 6-month history of urinary frequency, hesitancy and lower back pain.

840 A 4-year-old boy presents with a 3-week history of haematuria, fever and abdominal swelling. O/E: there is a palpable swelling in the left loin.

Theme: Bacterial infections

Options

    A. *Neisseria meningitidis*
    B. *Clostridium tetani*
    C. *Streptococcus pyogenes*
    D. *Staphylococcus aureus*
    E. *Klebsiella pneumoniae*
    F. *Escherichia coli*
    G. *Campylobacter jejuni*
    H. *Streptococcus pneumoniae*
    I. *Shigella sonnei*
    J. *Haemophilus influenzae*
    K. *Salmonella typhi*
    L. *Clostridium difficile*

Instructions

For each case, choose the single most appropriate organism from the list of options above. Each option may be used once, more than once or not at all.

841 A 63-year-old alcoholic presents with a 5-day history of fever, productive cough and shortness of breath. Chest X-ray shows right lower lobe consolidation. Sputum microscopy shows Gram-positive diplococci. Sputum culture shows the organism to be α-haemolytic.

842 A 34-year-old accountant presents with a 2-day history of vomiting and diarrhoea, following a meal at a restaurant. Stool microscopy shows Gram-negative motile rods.

843 A 24-year-old A&E nurse presents with severe headache, photophobia, fever and skin rash. Cerebrospinal fluid microscopy shows Gram-negative cocci.

844 A 69-year-old woman presents with dysuria and frequency of micturition for 3 days. Mid-stream urine microscopy shows Gram-negative bacilli.

845 A 23-year-old woman develops wound infection following an appendicectomy. Wound swab microscopy and culture shows Gram-positive, coagulase-positive cocci.

846 A 79-year-old woman who has had several courses of antibiotics for recurrent chest infections presents with worsening diarrhoea. Flexible sigmoidoscopy shows white mucosal plaques.

Theme: Earache

Options

A. Bell's palsy
B. Ramsay Hunt syndrome
C. Furunculosis
D. Carcinoma of the ear canal
E. Malignant otitis externa
F. Acute otitis externa
G. Acute otitis media
H. Bullous myringitis
I. Carcinoma of the tongue
J. Acute barotraumas
K. Rheumatoid arthritis
L. Cervical spondylosis

Instructions

For each case, choose the single most appropriate diagnosis from the list of options above. Each option may be used once, more than once or not at all.

847 A 74-year-old man who had been a heavy smoker for 50 years presents with a 2-month history of increasing left earache, painful tongue and impaired speech.

848 A 78-year-old man presents with a 3-week history of progressive right-side deafness, right LMNL VII palsy and bloodstained discharge from the right ear.

849 A 64-year-old secretary with a history of osteoporosis presents with pain and tenderness in the occipital region and around the right ear. She states that the pain is aggravated by neck movement.

850 An 8-year-old boy presents with severe left-side earache following recent flu. O/E: his temperature is 38.6°C, while his pulse is 120 bpm. Otoscopy shows a bulging and congested eardrum.

851 A 67-year-old man currently under treatment for lymphoma presents with acute onset left-side earache and left LMNL VII palsy. O/E: extremely tender vesicles in the left ear.

Theme: Differential diagnosis of ectopic pregnancy

Options

- A. Ectopic pregnancy
- B. Inevitable miscarriage
- C. Threatened miscarriage
- D. Endometriosis
- E. Missed abortion
- F. Pelvic inflammatory disease
- G. Septic abortion
- H. Ovarian cyst torsion
- I. Ureteric stone
- J. Appendicitis
- K. Crohn's disease
- L. Irritable bowel syndrome
- M. Cryptomenorrhoea

Instructions

For each case, choose the single most appropriate diagnosis from the list of options above. Each option may be used once, more than once or not at all.

852 A 17-year-old GCSE student presents 1 week before her exams having missed her period in addition to recurrent colicky abdominal pain and diarrhoea. General examination is normal, as are blood tests. Pregnancy test is negative.

853 A 28-year-old woman with an intrauterine contraceptive device, fitted 3 years ago, presents with a 2-month history of recurrent vaginal discharge and bleeding. Over the last 2 days, she developed lower abdominal pain and fever. Pregnancy test is negative.

854 A 24-year-old woman presents to A&E with severe lower abdominal pain and fresh vaginal bleeding. She admits to amenorrhoea for 10 weeks and a positive pregnancy test 3 weeks ago. O/E: abdominal tenderness and rigidity, bulky uterus and opened cervical os.

855 A 21-year-old student presents to A&E with severe left iliac fossa pain. Her last period was 3 weeks ago. An ultrasound shows a echogenic structure of 5 cm diameter in the left fornix.

856 A 27-year-old woman with a past history of pelvic inflammatory disease, and amenorrhoea for 8 weeks presents to A&E with left iliac fossa pain. She reports a small amount of brown watery vaginal discharge.

Theme: Infectious diseases

Options

- A. Candidiasis
- B. Hydatid cyst
- C. Giardiasis
- D. Amoebiasis
- E. Streptococcal pneumonia
- F. *Schistosoma mansoni* infection
- G. Toxoplasmosis
- H. Cryptosporidiosis
- I. *Plasmodium falciparum* malaria
- J. Strongyloidiasis
- K. *Pneumocystis jirovecii (carinii)* pneumonia
- L. Ovale malaria
- M. *Schistosoma haematobium* infection

Instructions

For each case, choose the single most appropriate diagnosis from the list of options above. Each option may be used once, more than once or not at all.

857 A 41-year-old businessman presents to his GP with fever and rigors 4 days after arrival from West Africa. He is prescribed antibiotics. Within 3 days, he presents to A&E with convulsions and dark urine. Examination reveals hepatosplenomegaly.

858 A 39-year-old Egyptian farmer with a history of rectal bleeding presents with haematemesis and weight loss. O/E: hepatosplenomegaly. Colonoscopy shows ulcers and polyps, particularly in the sigmoid colon and rectum.

859 A 29-year-old HIV-positive man presents with a 3-week history of dysphagia. Endoscopy shows white plaques in the oesophagus.

860 A 28-year-old woman presents with recurrent abdominal cramps and diarrhoea 2 weeks after returning from Southeast Asia. Colonoscopy shows multiple colonic ulcers. Biopsy shows PAS-positive trophozoites.

861 A 59-year-old man under treatment for leukaemia presents with dyspnoea on mild exertion and dry cough. Chest X-ray shows bilateral reticulonodular shadows. His oxygen saturation drops rapidly on exercise.

862 A 29-year-old butcher presents with mild fever, myalgia and maculopapular rash. O/E: mild hepatosplenomegaly and generalised lymphadenopathy.

Theme: DVLA regulations for Group 1 drivers

Options

A. Cases are considered on an individual basis.
B. Must not drive for at least 1 month. May resume driving if satisfactory recovery. DVLA need not be notified.
C. May resume driving once cerebral angiogram is normal and satisfactory recovery is achieved.
D. May resume driving only after a head CT scan is normal.
E. The licence must be refused or revoked.
F. Must not drive for 1 year. A short-period licence may be required thereafter.
G. May be allowed to drive if medical assessment confirms fitness to drive. A short-period licence may be required thereafter.
H. May resume driving only after an ETT is normal.
I. Must stop driving for at least 1 week. DVLA need not be notified.
J. Must stop driving for at least 4 weeks. DVLA need not be notified.
K. Driving may continue (unless treatment causes unacceptable side effects). DVLA need not be notified.
L. Must stop driving for 3 years, then reapply.
M. Must stop driving immediately, and for a minimum of 6 months.

Instructions

For each diagnosis, choose the single most appropriate course of action from the list of options above. Each option may be used once, more than once or not at all.

863 Simple faint with known provocation and prodromal symptoms
864 Angioplasty
865 Night blindness
866 Coronary artery bypass graft (CABG)
867 Cerebrovascular disease
868 Hypertension
869 First unprovoked epileptic seizure
870 Parkinson's disease
871 Migraine
872 Permanent pacemaker insertion

Theme: Scrotal swelling

Options

A. Testicular torsion
B. Inguinal hernia
C. Mumps orchitis
D. Sebaceous cyst
E. Testicular seminoma
F. Testicular teratoma
G. Epididymal cyst
H. Epididymo-orchitis
I. Tuberculous orchitis
J. Varicocele
K. Haematocele
L. Hydrocele

Instructions

For each case, choose the single most appropriate diagnosis from the list of options above. Each option may be used once, more than once or not at all.

873 A 19-year-old student presents with a 24-hour history of tender left scrotal swelling. He reported that it followed an injury during a game of rugby. O/E: the left hemiscrotum is very tender, fluctuant and does not transilluminate.

874 A healthy 63-year-old man presents with a 6-month history of a slowly enlarging scrotum. O/E: the left hemiscrotum is remarkably swollen, tense, non-tender but it transilluminates. The testis could not be felt and the neck of the scrotum is normal.

875 A 10-year-old boy presents at A&E with sudden-onset agonising right scrotal pain and vomiting. O/E: he is apyrexial, the scrotal skin is normal and the right testis is noted to be higher than the left. The patient refuses any further examination of the scrotum because of his pain.

876 A 27-year-old sailor presents with a 3-day history of worsening left scrotal pain, dysuria, urinary frequency and sweating. O/E: his temperature is 38.7°C, scrotal skin is red and hot and the left hemiscrotum is tender and swollen.

877 A 30-year-old man presents with a painless scrotal swelling. O/E: the right testis is slightly enlarged, hard in consistency and irregular in shape. Blood tests show remarkably elevated α-FP and β-HCG.

878 A 40-year-old man presents with a painless scrotal swelling. O/E: the right testis is enlarged, hard in consistency and irregular in shape. Blood tests show elevated β-HCG, while α-FP is normal.

Theme: Calcium and phosphate metabolism

Options

A. Primary hyperparathyroidism
B. Secondary hyperparathyroidism
C. Tertiary hyperparathyroidism
D. Paget's disease of bone
E. Hypoparathyroidism
F. Pseudohypoparathyroidism
G. Pseudopseudohypoparathyroidism
H. Multiple myeloma
I. Dietary vitamin D deficiency
J. Familial benign hypercalcaemia

Instructions

For each profile, choose the single most appropriate diagnosis from the list of options above. Each option may be used once, more than once or not at all.

879 Raised serum PTH, raised serum calcium, reduced serum phosphate, raised serum ALP, normal renal function and raised urinary calcium excretion.

880 Slightly raised serum PTH, reduced serum calcium, raised serum phosphate and normal renal function in a patient with short fourth and fifth metacarpal bones.

881 Normal serum PTH, normal serum calcium, normal serum phosphate, normal renal function and raised ALP.

882 Raised serum PTH, raised serum calcium, normal serum phosphate, raised serum ALP and impaired renal function.

883 Normal serum PTH, normal serum calcium, normal serum phosphate and normal renal function in a patient with short fourth and fifth metacarpal bones.

884 Raised serum PTH, low normal serum calcium, raised serum phosphate, impaired renal function and reduced vitamin D levels.

Theme: Investigating vaginal bleeding

Options

A. Full blood count
B. Gonadotrophin levels
C. Kleihauer–Betke test
D. Pregnancy test
E. Thyroid function test
F. Pituitary CT scan
G. Hysteroscopy
H. Transvaginal ultrasound scan
I. Endometrial sampling
J. Cervical inspection
K. Cervical smear
L. Endocervical swab
M. No investigations are necessary

Instructions

For each case, choose the single most appropriate investigation from the list of options above. Each option may be used once, more than once or not at all.

885 A 28-year-old woman with a 7-week history of amenorrhoea presents to her GP with severe right iliac fossa pain.

886 A 50-year-old woman on tamoxifen for breast cancer for 3 years presents with fresh vaginal bleeding. Her last period was 4 years ago. Her last cervical smear was 6 months ago and was normal.

887 A 46-year-old woman presents with a 4-month history of vaginal discharge and recurrent spotting. She had a normal cervical smear 5 years ago.

888 A 47-year-old woman presents with a 7-month history of irregular, prolonged but light periods. A pelvic ultrasound shows no abnormality.

889 A 23-year-old smoker is started on a combined oral contraceptive pill for the first time. She returns 2 months later complaining of intermenstrual bleeding.

Theme: Sexually transmitted diseases

Options

A. Chlamydia
B. Gonorrhoea
C. Syphilis
D. Lymphogranuloma venereum
E. Candidiasis
F. AIDS
G. Genital herpes simplex
H. Hepatitis B
I. Trichomoniasis
J. Chancroid
K. *Molluscum contagiosum*

Instructions

For each case, choose the single most appropriate diagnosis from the list of options above. Each option may be used once, more than once or not at all.

890 A 21-year-old student presents with a 10-day history of dysuria and white penile discharge. Microscopy of Gram-stained swabs showed diplococci.

891 A 24-year-old mechanic presents with a 2-week history of dysuria, watery penile discharge and testicular pain. Microscopy of Gram-stained swabs was negative.

892 A 35-year-old gay man presents with a 2-week history of anorectal pain, tenesmus and rectal discharge. Examination reveals tender inguinal lymphadenopathy.

893 A 28-year-old woman presents with severe vaginal itching and a yellow-green, frothy, foul-smelling vaginal discharge.

894 A 22-year-old man presents with multiple small painful ulcers on the penis. He reports that the lesions started as vesicles which crusted then ulcerated.

895 A 19-year-old student presents with three small pearly lesions on his penis. The lesions are painless, though they may bleed if scratched.

Theme: Electrolyte imbalance

Options

A. Conn's syndrome
B. Cushing's syndrome
C. Distal renal tubular acidosis
D. Proximal renal tubular acidosis
E. Pyloric stenosis
F. Addison's disease
G. Hyperosmolar non-ketotic coma (HONK)
H. Diabetic ketoacidosis (DKA)
I. Nephrogenic diabetes insipidus
J. Cranial diabetes insipidus
K. Liver cirrhosis
L. Gastrointestinal bleeding
M. Hepatorenal syndrome

Instructions

For each case, choose the single most appropriate diagnosis from the list of options above. Each option may be used once, more than once or not at all.

896 A 76-year-old woman is admitted via A&E after she collapsed at home. She has been unwell for 4 days and her GP diagnosed a viral illness. O/E: she is confused and her pulse is 130 bpm. Investigations: Hb 15.9 g/dL, WCC 12.3 × 10⁹/L, platelets 360 × 10⁹/L, urea 17.2 mmol/L, creatinine 145 μmol/L, Na 151 mmol/L, K 5.6 mmol/L, Cl 98 mmol/L, HCO₃ 22 mmol/L and glucose 64 mmol/L.

897 A 33-year-old man presents to his GP with a 3-month history of headache. O/E: blood pressure is 215/115 and fundoscopy shows grade 1 hypertensive retinopathy. Investigations: Na 148 mmol/L, K 3.1 mmol/L, urea 4.1 mmol/L, creatinine 98 μmol/L, HCO₃ 32 mmol/L and glucose 4.1 mmol/L. Urine dipstick is negative.

898 A 47-year-old man with a 5-year history of hepatitis C presents with shortness of breath and bilateral ankle swelling. O/E: blood pressure is 125/80, JVP is elevated (6 cm), bibasal crackles and mild ascites. Investigations: Na 132 mmol/L, K 3.5 mmol/L, urea 2.9 mmol/L, creatinine 90 μmol/L, HCO₃ 32 mmol/L, Cl 96 mmol/L, urinary Na < 10 mmol/L and urinary K 60 mmol/L.

899 A 22-year-old man presents with a 2-week history of recurrent loin pain. General examination is unremarkable. Investigations: Na 138 mmol/L, K 2.5 mmol/L, urea 3.8 mmol/L, creatinine 92 μmol/L, Cl 114 mmol/L, HCO₃ 15 mmol/L and urinary pH 6.5.

900 A 42-year-old woman with a long history of peptic ulcer presents with vomiting for 3 days. General examination is unremarkable. Investigations: Hb 16.2 g/dL, WCC 6.1 × 10⁹/L, platelets 330 × 10⁹/L, Na 138 mmol/L,

K 2.8 mmol/L, urea 14.3 mmol/L, creatinine 110 µmol/L, HCO_3 36 mmol/L, Cl 75 mmol/L and pH 7.52.

901 A 47-year-old woman with a history of pernicious anaemia and insulin-dependent diabetes mellitus presents with weight loss, fatigue, recurrent abdominal pain and darkening of skin. Investigations: Na 134 mmol/L, K 5.8 mmol/L, urea 8.2 mmol/L and creatinine 69 µmol/L.

Theme: Choice of analgesia

Options

- A. Paracetamol
- B. Morphine
- C. Tramadol
- D. Diclofenac
- E. Nitrous oxide
- F. Co-dydramol
- G. Diamorphine
- H. Gabapentin
- I. Ibuprofen
- J. Aspirin
- K. Pethidine
- L. Colchicine

Instructions

For each case, choose the single most appropriate analgesic from the list of options above. Each option may be used once, more than once or not at all.

902 A 16-year-old man dislocated the terminal phalanx of his right index finger while playing hockey. There is no fracture and analgesia is needed for reduction of the dislocation.

903 A 47-year-old woman complains of jaw pain following a dental extraction.

904 A 63-year-old woman complains of severe shooting pain in her right cheek and around her right eye following an attack of shingles.

905 A 74-year-old man with metastatic prostatic cancer presents with acute severe low backache. Simple analgesia was not effective.

906 A 70-year-old man presents with acutely painful, red, hot, swollen and tender left knee. He was recently started on diuretics by his GP. He has a history of gastritis.

907 A 40-year-old man presents with vomiting and acute abdominal pain. His amylase is 480 U/dL.

908 A 56-year-old man presents with acute chest pain. His ECG shows evidence of acute anterior myocardial infarction.

Theme: Dermatological cases

Options

A. Tinea corporis
B. Tinea versicolour
C. Meningococcal septicaemia
D. Dermatitis herpetiformis
E. Psoriasis
F. Atopic dermatitis
G. Shingles (herpes zoster)
H. Non-specific viral rash
I. Urticaria
J. Drug-induced rash
K. Scabies
L. Cutaneous larva migrans

Instructions

For each case, choose the single most appropriate diagnosis from the list of options above. Each option may be used once, more than once or not at all.

909 A 68-year-old man presents to his GP with pain, numbness and tingling adjacent to the right nipple and across the back. He is reassured and pre-scribed paracetamol. The next morning he develops a painful vesicular rash across the same distribution.

910 A 25-year-old fitness instructor presents with a 4-week history of spreading and itchy pink plaques with raised scaly edges.

911 A 32-year-old woman is brought to A&E unconscious. On examination she is pyrexial, and has purple rash which does not blanch on pressure.

912 A 27-year-old man presents to his GP with a few white oval spots on the chest and back, covered by thin scales. He was advised to try skin emol-lients. After returning from holiday 4 weeks later, he was distressed as the lesions failed to resolve and became more obvious as they failed to tan.

913 A 27-year-old woman presents with pruritic papules, plaques and vesicles on the extensor surfaces of the arms, knees and buttocks. On further questioning, she reports bloating and weight loss for 4 months.

914 A 15-month-old toddler is brought by her mother to A&E as she was pyrexial and had a skin rash. On examination her temperature was 38°C and there was a widespread maculopapular rash on the trunk. She had a runny nose and mild cervical lymphadenopathy but her chest was clear.

Theme: Causes of mouth ulcers

Options

A. Ulcerative colitis
B. Crohn's disease
C. Behçet's disease
D. Reiter's syndrome
E. Varicella zoster virus
F. Herpes simplex
G. Syphilis
H. Aphthous ulcers
I. Systemic lupus erythematosus
J. Squamous cell carcinoma
K. Lichen planus
L. Stevens–Johnson syndrome

Instructions

For each case, choose the single most appropriate diagnosis from the list of options above. Each option may be used once, more than once or not at all.

915 A 33-year-old woman is admitted via A&E feeling extremely unwell. O/E: she is pyrexial with a temperature of 38.7°C. There are target-like lesions on her arms and legs and severe oral ulceration with crusts. She was recently started on an antibiotic for a chest infection.

916 A 32-year-old Cypriot man with a past medical history of deep venous thrombosis, uveitis and arthritis presents with recurrent orogenital ulcers.

917 A 59-year-old man currently on treatment for lymphoma presents with severe pain and reduced vision in his right eye. O/E: periocular and corneal vesicles.

918 A 27-year-old sailor presents to his GP with a large painless indurated ulcer in his tongue. It started 2 weeks earlier as a small papule.

919 A 13-year-old boy, normally fit and well, presents with a 6-month history of multiple painful oral ulcers which heal spontaneously within 2–8 weeks.

920 A 37-year-old woman with a history of diarrhoea, weight loss, rectal bleeding and perianal fistula presents with two painful buccal ulcers.

Theme: Abdominal discomfort

Options

A. Endometriosis
B. Irritable bowel syndrome
C. Pelvic inflammatory disease
D. Inflammatory bowel disease
E. Endometrial carcinoma
F. Acute appendicitis
G. Ovarian carcinoma
H. Ruptured ovarian cyst
I. Torsion of an ovarian cyst
J. Colonic carcinoma
K. Mesenteric adenitis
L. Diverticulitis

Instructions

For each case, choose the single most appropriate diagnosis from the list of options above. Each option may be used once, more than once or not at all.

921 A 29-year-old smoker presents with a 6-month history of recurrent abdominal pain with intermittent diarrhoea and constipation. She denies any rectal bleeding. Her periods are regular. Abdominal ultrasound and colonoscopy are normal. Vaginal and cervical swabs are negative.

922 A 54-year-old woman presents with constipation and weight loss, while feeling an increase in abdominal girth. She admits to bloating after meals. She denies any rectal bleeding. Colonoscopy is normal.

923 A 14-year-old virgin presents at mid-cycle with severe acute right-side lower abdominal pain which resolves within 8 hours. She is apyrexial and all her blood results are normal.

924 A 22-year-old smoker presents with a 3-month history of abdominal discomfort and weight loss of 5 kg. She also admits to three episodes of fresh rectal bleeding where the blood was mixed with stools. O/E: raised tender oval lesions over both shins.

925 A 26-year-old woman who was previously treated for chlamydial urethritis presents with lower abdominal pain and fever. O/E: diffuse lower abdominal tenderness, positive cervical excitation test and adnexal tenderness.

926 A 79-year-old woman with a long history of constipation presents with fever, left iliac fossa pain, nausea and loss of appetite. O/E: tenderness and rigidity in the left iliac fossa. Rectal examination was very painful and showed hard stools.

Theme: Medical syndromes

Options

- A. Down's syndrome
- B. Turner's syndrome
- C. Klinefelter's syndrome
- D. Sheehan's syndrome
- E. Eaton–Lambert syndrome
- F. Antiphospholipid syndrome
- G. Neuroleptic malignant syndrome
- H. Guillain–Barré syndrome
- I. McArdle's disease
- J. Goodpasture's syndrome
- K. Churg–Strauss syndrome
- L. Reiter's syndrome

Instructions

For each case, choose the single most appropriate diagnosis from the list of options above. Each option may be used once, more than once or not at all.

927 A 32-year-old psychotic patient is admitted via A&E with rigidity and fever. His blood results show significantly elevated creatinine phosphokinase and renal impairment.

928 A 43-year-old man with a recent history of gastroenteritis presents with increasing weakness of his legs and right arm associated with numbness and tingling. O/E: absent tendon reflexes. No sensory level is detected.

929 A 16-year-old woman presents to her GP with primary amenorrhoea. O/E: her height is 143 cm, with bilateral ptosis, high arched palate, cubitus vulgus and swelling of both ankles.

930 A 69-year-old man with recently diagnosed small cell (oat cell) carcinoma of the lung presents with weakness and easy fatiguability. O/E: proximal muscle weakness, particularly in lower limbs, and reduced tendon reflexes.

931 A 30-year-old man is investigated for infertility. O/E: his height is 194 cm, with gynaecomastia and very small testes.

932 A 38-year-old businessman presents with dysuria, sore eyes and buccal ulceration 1 month after returning from a trip to the Far East. He reports having had a venereal infection after his return.

933 A 32-year-old woman is admitted with deep venous thrombosis for the third time in 1 year. She has a past history of a transient ischaemic attack, migraine, epilepsy and three miscarriages.

Theme: Seizures

Options

A. Hyponatraemia
B. Hypocalcaemia
C. Hypomagnesaemia
D. Meningitis
E. Cerebral abscess
F. Subdural haematoma
G. Tonic–clonic seizure
H. Complex partial seizure
I. Simple partial seizure
J. Partial seizure with secondary generalisation
K. Atonic seizure
L. Typical absence seizure

Instructions

For each case, choose the single most appropriate diagnosis from the list of options above. Each option may be used once, more than once or not at all.

934 A 17-year-old student is brought to A&E after she had a witnessed fit. History was given by a friend as she was too drowsy. She suddenly lost consciousness while sitting on a sofa, fell to the floor, then became rigid and started shaking all limbs vigorously. She bit her tongue and was incontinent of urine.

935 A 70-year-old man under palliative treatment for bronchogenic carcinoma is prescribed a diuretic for ankle oedema. Over the next 10 days he becomes more confused, then he develops a tonic–clonic seizure.

936 A 7-year-old girl is reported by her teachers as developing several 'funny turns' during which she becomes vague and stops whatever she is doing for a few seconds, then continues again as if nothing has happened.

937 A 14-year-old girl is referred to neurologists after having four fits in 3 weeks. It always starts by feeling vague (but conscious), which is followed by a phase of anxiety and apprehension. She then collapses, loses her consciousness and starts shaking, which is associated with biting of the tongue and urinary incontinence.

938 A 49-year-old woman develops a tonic–clonic seizure while on a surgical ward 1 day after a thyroidectomy.

939 A 23-year-old woman who is 10 weeks pregnant with a 3-week history of hyperemesis gravidarum is brought to A&E after she collapsed and started fitting.

Theme: Red eyes

Options

A. Herpetic corneal ulcer
B. Scleritis
C. Allergic conjunctivitis
D. Bacterial conjunctivitis
E. Viral conjunctivitis
F. Anterior uveitis
G. Pterygium
H. Acute closed-angle glaucoma
I. Subconjunctival haemorrhage
J. Open-angle glaucoma
K. Episcleritis
L. Trachoma

Instructions

For each case, choose the single most appropriate diagnosis from the list of options above. Each option may be used once, more than once or not at all.

940 A 6-year-old child recovering from whooping cough presents with sudden-onset painless and red left eye.

941 A 39-year-old man recently diagnosed with Behçet's disease presents with a 3-month history of recurrent photophobia, reduced visual acuity and watery red eyes.

942 A 31-year-old nurse presents with a 2-day history of photophobia, reduced visual acuity and severe pain in the right eye. O/E: red and watery right eye. Fluorescin eye drops show a dendritic corneal ulcer.

943 A 62-year-old man presents to A&E with acute severe pain in the left eye with impaired vision and haloes around light. The pain started while he was at the cinema. He vomited twice while waiting in A&E.

944 A 3-year-old child woke up with purulent discharge and discomfort in both eyes. His vision is intact. O/E: the conjunctivae are inflamed bilaterally.

945 A 12-year-old child from the Middle East is referred to an ophthalmology clinic with entropion and trichiasis. O/E: corneal scar and upper-lid conjunctivae shows cobblestone appearance.

946 A 60-year-old chemical engineer who worked in the Middle Eastern oil fields for 18 years presents with a 9-month history of progressive encroachment of the conjunctivae over the cornea. His vision is still intact.

Theme: Thoracic tumours

Options

A. Neurofibroma
B. Germ cell tumour
C. Pulmonary metastases
D. Hodgkin's lymphoma
E. Squamous cell carcinoma of the bronchus
F. Adenocarcinoma of the bronchus
G. Carcinoid tumour
H. Small cell (oat cell) carcinoma of the bronchus
I. Leiomyosarcoma of the lung
J. Thymoma
K. Oesophageal carcinoma
L. Pleural mesothelioma

Instructions

For each case, choose the single most appropriate diagnosis from the list of options above. Each option may be used once, more than once or not at all.

947 A 74-year-old heavy smoker presents with a 4-month history of weight loss, tiredness, lethargy and recently haemoptysis. Blood tests show hypokalaemia.

948 A 45-year-old woman with a long history of myasthenia gravis presents with a 6-week history of dysphagia mainly to solids. Lateral view chest X-ray shows an anterior mediastinal mass.

949 A 72-year-old retired underground train driver presents with a 4-month history of weight loss and worsening shortness of breath. Chest X-ray shows diffuse pleural thickening at the right lung base.

950 A 48-year-old man presents with a 3-month history of weight loss, night fever and sweating. O/E: bilateral palpable axillary and cervical lymphadenopathy. Chest X-ray shows a mediastinal shadow.

951 A 62-year-old Chinese woman who has never smoked presents with weight loss and general deterioration of health. Abdominal ultrasound shows liver metastases. Chest X-ray shows a 3-cm shadow in the right lower lobe. Bronchoscopy is normal.

952 A 67-year-old heavy smoker is admitted with acute renal impairment. It is noted that his corrected calcium is 3.09 mmol/L. A chest X-ray shows a 2-cm shadow in the middle zone of the right lung.

Theme: Headache

Options

    A. Bacterial meningitis
    B. Cervical spondylosis
    C. Migraine
    D. Idiopathic (benign) intracranial hypertension
    E. Subarachnoid haemorrhage
    F. Extradural haemorrhage
    G. Meningioma
    H. Cluster headache
    I. Subdural haematoma
    J. Trigeminal neuralgia
    K. Giant cell arteritis
    L. Tension headache
    M. Viral meningitis

Instructions

For each case, choose the single most appropriate diagnosis from the list of options above. Each option may be used once, more than once or not at all.

953 A 19-year-old soldier presents with severe headache, fever, photophobia and widespread blotchy skin rash.

954 A 74-year-old man presents with frontal headache, pain on jaw movement and weight loss. He had had a similar problem 3 years earlier which had responded to prednisolone. Temporal artery biopsy is normal.

955 A 27-year-old athlete presents with a sudden onset of severe headache associated with nausea and vomiting. O/E: GCS is 8/15 and he has marked neck stiffness. He is apyrexial. Fundoscopy reveals subhyaloid haemorrhage.

956 A 41-year-old lawyer presents with a 3-month history of recurrent headaches which feel like a tight band around the head.

957 A 49-year-old man presents with a 4-week history of recurrent headaches occurring at the same time every day, shortly after going to sleep. It is usually associated with pain around the right eye and lacrimation. There is no aura and each episode lasts less than an hour. The headache is relieved by movement rather than by remaining still.

958 A 24-year-old obese woman on oral contraceptive pills presents with a 3-month history of morning headaches which are aggravated by coughing, sneezing or straining. She has also noted occasional blurring of vision. Fundoscopy shows bilateral papilloedema.

959 A 36-year-old woman presents with a 2-month history of recurrent severe right-side headaches associated with vomiting and blurring of vision. She feels generally unwell, lethargic and nauseated about 12–24 hours before each episode.

Theme: Vaginal bleeding

Options

A. Endometrial carcinoma
B. Foreign body
C. Ectopic pregnancy
D. Atrophic vaginitis
E. Bleeding disorder
F. Cervical ectropion
G. Endometriosis
H. Cervical carcinoma
I. Cervical polyp
J. Normal menstruation
K. Miscarriage (spontaneous abortion)
L. Threatened abortion

Instructions

For each case, choose the single most appropriate diagnosis from the list of options above. Each option may be used once, more than once or not at all.

960 A 62-year-old woman presents with post-coital bleeding, dyspareunia and urinary stress incontinence.

961 A 71-year-old psychiatric patient presents with a 3-week history of progressive vaginal bleeding and offensive discharge. She is otherwise fit. Speculum examination is diagnostic.

962 A 27-year-old woman presents with a very heavy period and passes several blood clots. Her last period was 56 days ago. Her periods are usually light and regular. She is otherwise fit and healthy.

963 A 37-year-old woman with a history of pelvic inflammatory disease and metrorrhagia presents with dark vaginal bleeding and a 2-day history of colicky right iliac fossa pain.

964 A 59-year-old obese woman presents with postmenopausal bleeding. She had regular periods until 3 years ago. General and speculum examination reveal no abnormality. Vaginal ultrasound shows endometrial thickening.

965 A 40-year-old woman presents with a 4-week history of post-coital bleeding. Speculum examination shows a cervical ulcer. An endocervical smear shows dyskaryosis.

966 A 34-year-old woman presents with a 5-month history of menorrhagia. Diagnosis is confirmed by laparoscopy.

967 A 28-year-old woman on combined oral contraceptive pills presents with a 3-month history of post-coital and intermenstrual bleeding. Speculum examination shows an everted ulcerated cervix. An endocervial smear is normal.

Theme: Investigating a neck swelling

Options

    A. Thyroid function test
    B. Excision biopsy
    C. Digital subtraction angiography
    D. Sialogram
    E. Ultrasound
    F. Direct nasopharyngoscopy
    G. Technetium scan
    H. Paul–Bunnell test
    I. Doppler ultrasound
    J. Fine-needle aspiration
    K. Full blood count
    L. Iodine uptake scan

Instructions

For each case, choose the single most appropriate investigation from the list of options above. Each option may be used once, more than once or not at all.

968 A 60-year-old woman presents with an 8-month history of a slowly growing mass below the left angle of the jaw. O/E: the swelling is painless, mobile and firm. There is no evidence of VII palsy or any neurological deficit.

969 A 77-year-old alcoholic and heavy smoker presents with a 6-week history of hoarseness of voice. O/E: there is a hard painless swelling in the anterior triangle of the neck.

970 A 30-year-old fit mechanic presents with a 3-week history of intermittent painful swelling below his jaw. The pain and swelling are worse on eating. O/E: there is a little tender swelling in the right submandibular region.

971 A 74-year-old hypertensive man presents with a neck swelling which has increased in size over the last 4 months. O/E: there is a pulsatile swelling in the anterior triangle of the neck. There is a bruit on auscultation.

972 A 50-year-old woman presents with a 3-month history of a neck swelling and hoarse voice. O/E: there is a multinodular goitre but she is clinically euthyroid.

973 A 42-year-old fit woman presents with a 4-month history of a neck swelling. O/E: there is a palpable painless solitary thyroid nodule. She is clinically euthyroid.

Theme: Abdominal pain

Options

A. Acute myocardial infarction
B. Gastro-oesophageal reflux disease
C. Acute pancreatitis
D. Ruptured abdominal aortic aneurysm
E. Colonic carcinoma
F. Acute appendicitis
G. Ascending cholangitis
H. Crohn's disease
I. Sickle cell crisis
J. Acute cholecystitis
K. Mesenteric vascular occlusion
L. Acute ureteric colic

Instructions

For each case, choose the single most appropriate diagnosis from the list of options above. Each option may be used once, more than once or not at all.

974 A 21-year-old woman, normally fit and healthy, presents with a 12-hour history of severe right iliac fossa pain, nausea and vomiting. O/E: guarding rigidity and rebound tenderness in the right iliac fossa.

975 A 47-year-old alcoholic presents with a 24-hour history of severe epigastric pain radiating to the back, nausea and vomiting. O/E: epigastric tenderness and rigidity. Investigations show macrocytic anaemia, leucocytosis, hyperglycaemia and prolonged clotting.

976 A 49-year-old obese woman presents with a 48-hour history of fever, rigors and right upper quadrant pain. O/E: jaundice. Full blood count shows leucocytosis. Abdominal X-ray shows gas in the biliary tree.

977 A 67-year-old heavy smoker presents with a 7-hour history of severe epigastric pain, nausea and palpitations. Abdominal X-ray is normal as well as full blood count, liver function tests and urea and electrolytes. Creatinine phosphokinase is markedly raised.

978 A 76-year-old hypertensive smoker with a 4-month history of backache presents with acute excruciating epigastric pain radiating to the back. O/E: blood pressure is 85/50 mmHg, pulse is 130 bpm (right femoral pulse is absent, while left femoral pulse is weak), marked abdominal tenderness and rigidity.

Theme: Prescribing antimicrobials

Options

- A. Piperacillin
- B. Trimethoprim
- C. Augmentin and clarithromycin
- D. Augmentin
- E. Acyclovir
- F. Fluconazole
- G. Amoxycillin and clarithromycin and omeprazole
- H. Metronidazole
- I. Clotrimazole
- J. Amphotericin B
- K. Flucloxacillin
- L. Rifampicin

Instructions

For each infection, choose the single most appropriate antimicrobial from the list of options above. Each option may be used once, more than once or not at all.

979 *Helicobacter pylori*

980 Oesophageal candidiasis

981 *Pseudomonas* wound infection

982 Community-acquired pneumonia in an elderly man with heart failure.

983 Aspergillosis

984 Amoebiasis

985 Vaginal candidiasis

986 Herpes labialis

Theme: Liver disease

Options

A. Alcoholic liver disease
B. Primary biliary cirrhosis
C. Gallstones
D. Wilson's disease
E. Hepatitis B
F. Portal vein thrombosis
G. Carcinoma of the head of pancreas
H. Gilbert's syndrome
I. Haemochromatosis
J. Metastatic liver disease
K. Autoimmune liver disease
L. Budd–Chiari syndrome

Instructions

For each case, choose the single most appropriate diagnosis from the list of options above. Each option may be used once, more than once or not at all.

987 A 38-year-old woman on oral contraceptive pills presents with progressive jaundice and right-upper quadrant pain. She has a history of deep venous thrombosis. O/E: tender hepatomegaly, ascites, bilateral ankle and sacral oedema. The spleen was not palpable.

988 A 62-year-old man presents with a 3-week history of progressive jaundice, dark urine, plate stools and weight loss of 6 kg. O/E: jaundice, but no organomegaly or ascites. Abdominal ultrasound confirms a dilated common bile duct and gall bladder, but no gallstones are seen. The pancreas could not be visualised clearly due to bowel gas.

989 A 36-year-old man presents with a 3-day history of fever, productive cough and shortness of breath. O/E: jaundice, but no organomegaly or ascites. Chest auscultation reveals few left basal crackles. Chest X-ray shows left-lower lobe consolidation. Liver function tests are normal apart from unconjugated hyperbilirubinaemia.

990 A 47-year-old woman presents with a 5-week history of worsening jaundice and a 3-month history of severe itching which did not respond to antihistamines. O/E: 2-cm hepatomegaly, clubbing, xanthomata and jaundice.

991 A 57-year-old man with a history of arthritis, diabetes mellitus and congestive cardiac failure noted that his skin had become darker and that he had become more lethargic recently. O/E: 1-cm hepatomegaly, 1-cm splenomegaly and gynaecomastia.

Theme: Carcinogens

Options

A. Nitrosamines
B. Ultraviolet light
C. Human herpes virus type 8
D. Aflatoxin B_1
E. Epstein–Barr virus
F. Polycyclic aromatic hydrocarbons
G. Human papilloma virus
H. β-naphthylamine
I. Betel nut
J. Arsenic
K. Asbestos
L. Ionising radiation
M. Benzene

Instructions

For each tumour, choose the single most appropriate carcinogen from the list of options above. Each option may be used once, more than once or not at all.

992 Hepatocellular carcinoma
993 Adenocarcinoma of the stomach
994 Oral cancer
995 Leukaemia
996 Transitional cell carcinoma of the bladder
997 Kaposi's sarcoma
998 Malignant melanoma of the skin
999 Squamous cell carcinoma of the cervix
1000 Burkitt's lymphoma

Answers

1 G HRT is a risk factor for deep vein thrombosis (DVT), which can then result in pulmonary embolism.

2 J Pleural effusion has a characteristic shadow on the CXR, rising towards the axilla.

3 K Clubbing and bilateral inspiratory crackles typically point towards CFA, particularly if the patient is above 50 years old.

4 E EAA is more common in specific occupations, e.g. farmers, ventilation system workers and vets. It can present as an acute, subacute or chronic form.

5 F Primary spontaneous pneumothorax tends to occur in young people without underlying lung problems, though it is more common in tall male smokers.

6 C A classic sign of pulmonary oedema is the production of pink frothy sputum. A normal Doppler excludes DVT. The presence of a third heart sound is predictive of cardiogenic pulmonary oedema.

7 D Hereditary haemochromatosis is an autosomal recessive disease with estimated prevalence in the population of 0.2% in Caucasians. The gene responsible for hereditary haemochromatosis (known as *HFE* gene) is located on chromosome 6.

8 I HCC most commonly appears in a patient with chronic viral hepatitis B or C and/or alcoholics with cirrhosis.

9 B PSC is closely linked with ulcerative colitis. The definitive treatment is liver transplantation.

10 K Chronic active hepatitis, or autoimmune hepatitis occurs in adults and children, with two peaks of incidence at age 10–20 years and again at age 45–70 years. Systemic or cutaneous abnormalities occur in 25% of patients.

11 E Galactosaemia is not related to and should not be confused with lactose intolerance. It follows an autosomal recessive mode of inheritance.

12 G Dubin–Johnson syndrome is an autosomal recessive disorder that causes an increase of conjugated bilirubin without elevation of liver enzymes (ALT, AST). This condition is associated with a defect in the ability of hepatocytes to secrete conjugated bilirubin into the bile. It is usually asymptomatic.

13 D Oesophageal varices are most often a consequence of portal hypertension, commonly due to cirrhosis.

14 G Dysphagia to solids always requires urgent referral to exclude oesophageal cancer.

15 E Those are typical features of gastric cancer.

16 F Crohn's disease may affect any part of the gastrointestinal tract from mouth to anus. It is associated with seronegative spondyloarthropathy.

17 C Mallory–Weiss syndrome refers to bleeding from tears in the mucosa at the junction of the stomach and oesophagus, usually caused by severe retching, coughing or vomiting.

18 A Duodenal ulcer is characterised by pain mostly before meals or when hungry. It may be eased by food.

19 D Hypertension is a risk factor for brainstem haemorrhage. Nystagmus, vertigo and incoordination point towards brainstem/cerebellar pathology.

20 A Subdural haematoma may be acute, subacute or chronic. Loss of consciousness or fluctuating levels of consciousness is a common feature.

21 G Idiopathic intracranial hypertension is defined as raised intracranial pressure in the absence of a mass lesion or of hydrocephalus. The condition appears to be due to impaired cerebrospinal fluid absorption from the subarachnoid space across the arachnoid villi into the dural sinuses. Prompt recognition and treatment are needed to prevent potentially permanent visual loss. It is most frequently occurs in obese women of childbearing age.

22 F Multiple sclerosis takes several forms, with new symptoms occurring either in discrete attacks (relapsing forms) or slowly accumulating over time (progressive forms). Between attacks, symptoms may fully resolve, but permanent neurological problems often occur, especially as the disease advances.

23 I In practice, fever, headache and rash means meningitis until proven otherwise.

24 B Guillain–Barré syndrome is an acute inflammatory demyelinating polyneuropathy. Ascending paralysis, weakness beginning in the feet and hands and migrating towards the trunk, is the most typical symptom. The disease is usually triggered by an acute infection.

25 B Weight loss, mild anaemia, fever and raised ESR all point to TB.

26 F Lymphoma is characterised by painless lymphadenopathy which becomes painful after alcohol consumption.

27 E Caecal carcinoma typically presents with unexplained pain in the right iliac fossa plus or minus general symptoms such as anaemia, malaise and weakness. Abdominal pain often develops late in the disease because the tumour may remain silent until it has grown to a considerable size. Commonly the condition is seen in 70- to 80-year-olds. Women are more affected than men.

28 G An ectopic kidney is typically asymptomatic.

29 C String sign represents a severe narrowing of loop of bowel, in which a thin stripe of contrast within the lumen looks like a string. It may be seen in Crohn's disease, hypertrophic pyloric stenosis, carcinoid and colon cancer.

30 B Anorexia nervosa patients are usually young, with low self-esteem and suffering from stress. There is typically a disturbed body image, where they feel they are overweight despite being extremely underweight. Amenorrhoea for 3 months or more is very common. Bulimia nervosa on the other hand is characterised by restraining of food intake followed by binge eating, which is typically complicated by guilt feelings resulting in induced vomiting and abuse of laxatives and diuretics.

31 G ESR in men < 50 is < 15 mm/h and in women in the same age group < 20 mm/h. The normal result for men > 50 is < 20 mm/h and in women in the same age group < 30 mm/h. A normal FBC makes leukaemia unlikely while a normal bone profile makes multiple myeloma unlikely.

32 H The age distribution of patients with coeliac disease is bimodal, the first at 8–12 months and the second in the third to fourth decades. The bulky, greasy appearance and rancid odor of stools often suggest malabsorption of fat, which is a feature of coeliac disease. Absence of rectal bleeding or mucous excludes ulcerative colitis.

33 F Presentating with polydipsia and polyuria should always raise suspicion of diabetes mellitus, diabetes insipidus or hypercalcaemia. Hypercalcaemia in an elderly male smoker should alert to the possibility of a non-small cell lung cancer (specifically squamous cell carcinoma).

34 G *Pneumocystis* is commonly found in the lungs of healthy people, but being a source of opportunistic infection it can cause a lung infection in people with a weak immune system. *Pneumocystis* pneumonia is especially seen in people with cancer, HIV/AIDS, and when the use of medications affect the immune system. The older name *Pneumocystis carinii* (which now only applies to the *Pneumocystis* variant that occurs in animals) is still in common usage.

35 D Patients with Legionnaires' disease usually have fever, chills, and a cough, which may be dry or may produce sputum. Some patients also have muscle aches, headache, tiredness, loss of appetite, loss of coordination (ataxia), and occasionally diarrhoea and vomiting.

36 F *Mycoplasma pneumoniae* is called atypical pneumonia because of its protracted course, lack of sputum production and wealth of extra-pulmonary symptoms.

37 H Psittacosis is an infection caused by *Chlamydophila psittaci*, a type of bacteria found in the droppings of birds. Doxycycline is the first line treatment.

38 A Multiple abscesses point to an *S. aureus* infection.

39 J About 60% of people with cystic fibrosis have a chronic respiratory infection caused by *Pseudomonas aeruginosa* that settles into the thick mucus trapped in the airways. Once it settles in the respiratory tract, it is hard to get rid of. Respiratory failure caused by the infection is often the ultimate cause of death in many people with CF.

40 D Exposure to radiation is a risk factor for aplastic anaemia.

41 J Phenytoin causes a reduction in folic acid levels. Folic acid is presented in foods as polyglutamate, which is then converted into monoglutamates by intestinal conjugase. Phenytoin acts by inhibiting this enzyme, thereby causing folate deficiency.

42 B Spherocytosis is an auto-haemolytic anaemia, characterised by the production of erythrocytes that are sphere shaped. Spherocytes are found in hereditary spherocytosis and autoimmune haemolytic anaemia. The misshapen but otherwise healthy erythrocytes are mistaken by the spleen for old or damaged erythrocytes and it thus constantly breaks them down, causing auto-haemolysis.

43 C Types of AIHA include warm autoimmune haemolytic anaemia, cold agglutinin disease and paroxysmal cold haemoglobinuria. AIHA can be induced by several drugs, e.g. methyldopa, and also by some disease conditions, including *Mycoplasma pneumoniae* and infectious mononucleosis.

44 H Thalassaemia is an inherited autosomal recessive disease. The genetic defect, which could be either mutation or deletion, results in reduced rate of synthesis or no synthesis of one of the globin chains that make up haemoglobin. This can cause the formation of abnormal haemoglobin molecules, thus causing anaemia.

45 I G6PD deficiency is the most common human enzyme defect. It is an X-linked recessive hereditary disease.

46 A Subungal hyperkeratosis is typical of psoriasis, which can also cause transverse or longitudinal ridging.

47 J Beau's lines are single transverse ridges affecting all nails due to an acute systemic illness affecting the growth of all nails. They move distally with nail growth over a period of a few months.

48 F Lichen planus is characterised by nail plate thinning and longitudinal ridging.

49 D Onychogryphosis is a hypertrophy that may produce nails resembling claws. It is usually secondary to neglect and failure to cut the nails for extended periods of time.

50 G Koilonychia (spoon nails) is a nail disease that may be a sign of iron deficiency anaemia.

51 M Brown or black linear streaks may be due to melanoma, particularly if expanding and showing variation in shape and colour.

52 H Arrhenoblastoma is a rare tumour. It accounts for less than 0.5% of all ovarian tumours. These tumours are found in women of all age groups, but are most common in young women.

53 A Mucinous cystadenoma is the most common large ovarian tumour. It is filled with mucinous material and rupture may cause pseudomyxoma peritonei. It may be multilocular. It is most common in the 30–50 age group. About 5% will be malignant.

54 F Serous cystadenoma is most common in women aged between 30–40 years. Thirty per cent are bilateral and about 30% are malignant.

55 I Benign ovarian fibroma can be left alone when it is not causing the patient any trouble. When symptomatic, laparoscopic surgery is frequently performed to remove an ovarian fibroma.

56 D A teratoma is an encapsulated tumour with tissue or organ components resembling normal derivatives of all three germ layers.

57 J Granulosa-theca cell tumours account for approximately 2% of all ovarian tumours and can be divided into adult (95%) and juvenile (5%) types based on histological findings.

58 G Cystic fibrosis can be diagnosed before birth by genetic testing, or by a sweat test in early childhood.

59 A Recurrent right hypochondrial pain in a female above 40 points to gallstones.

60 E Diagnosing polyarteritis nodosa is supported by tests that indicate inflammation, including elevation of blood sedimentation rate and C-reactive protein. The white blood cell count and platelet count can be elevated, while the red blood count is decreased. Hepatitis B virus testing can be positive in 10%–20% of patients with polyarteritis nodosa. Urine testing can show protein and red blood cells. The diagnosis is confirmed by a biopsy of involved tissue that reveals vasculitis.

61 H Painless jaundice occurs when cancer of the head of the pancreas (about 60% of cases) obstructs the common bile duct. Carcinoma of the body or tail of the pancreas is typically associated with epigastric pain radiating to the back.

62 K There is a general mnemonic for remembering the effects of hypercalcaemia: 'groans (constipation), moans (e.g. fatigue, lethargy and depression), bones (bone pain, especially if PTH is elevated), stones (kidney stones) and psychiatric overtones (including depression and confusion)'.

63 C Pancreatitis occurs in about 4% of mumps cases, manifesting as abdominal pain and vomiting.

64 D About 50% of cases of aortic stenosis are due to age-related calcification of the normal trileaflet valve. Other predisposing conditions include calcification of a congenital bicuspid aortic valve (30%–40% of cases) and acute rheumatic fever (< 10% of cases).

65 H About 50% of cases of aortic regurgitation are due to aortic root dilatation, which is idiopathic in >80% of cases.

66 E HCM is frequently asymptomatic until sudden cardiac death. Its prevalence is about 0.4% of the general population.

67 A Almost all cases of mitral stenosis are secondary to rheumatic fever. The normal area of the mitral valve orifice is about 4–6 cm².

68 F Mitral regurgitation is the most common form of valvular heart disease. It has an incidence of approximately 2% of the population, affecting males and females equally.

69 K The ventricular septum consists of an inferior muscular and superior membranous portion. Congenital ventral septal defects are the most common congenital heart defects.

70 G Chickenpox is due to primary infection with varicella zoster virus. It usually starts with vesicular skin rash, mainly on the body and head rather than at the periphery, and becomes itchy, raw pockmarks, which mostly heal without scarring. It is an airborne disease spread easily through coughing or sneezing, or through direct contact with secretions from the rash. A person with chickenpox is infectious from 1–5 days before the rash appears. The contagious period continues for 4–5 days after the appearance of the rash, or until all lesions have crusted over.

71 F Erythema infectiosum or fifth disease is one of several possible manifestations of infection by erythrovirus (previously called parvovirus B19). The disease is also referred to as slapped cheek syndrome. Bright red cheeks are a defining symptom of the infection in children.

72 A Itchy rash in the folds between fingers is characteristic of scabies.

73 D Rubella is often mild and attacks often pass unnoticed. It can last 1–3 days. Children recover more quickly than adults. Lymphadenopathy can persist for up to a week and the fever rarely rises above 38°C.

74 B Measles spreads through respiration (contact with fluids from an infected person's nose and mouth, either directly or through aerosol transmission), and is highly contagious. It has an average incubation period of 14 days (range 6–19 days), and infectivity lasts from 2–4 days prior until 2–5 days following the onset of the rash.

75 K In clinical practice, fever and peticheal rash means meningitis until proved otherwise.

76 A The term 'melanotic stools' is sometimes used to refer to black, tarry stools or blood in stools. Meckel's diverticulum is a pouch on the wall of the lower part of the intestine that is present at birth (congenital). The diverticulum may contain tissue that is identical to tissue of the stomach or pancreas. Approximately 2% of the population has a Meckel's diverticulum, but only a few people develop symptoms (abdominal pain and/or rectal bleeding).

77 D Haemolytic–uraemic syndrome is a disease characterised by haemolytic anaemia, acute renal failure and a low platelet count. It predominantly but not exclusively affects children. Most cases are preceded by an episode of diarrhoea caused by *E. coli*, which is acquired as a food-borne illness. It is a medical emergency and carries a 5%–10% mortality; of the remainder, the majority recover without major consequences, but a small proportion develop chronic kidney disease and become reliant on renal replacement therapy.

78 B Eosinophilic colitis is characterised by eosinophilic infiltration localised only in the large bowel, resulting in fever, diarrhoea, bloody stools, constipation, obstruction/strictures, acute abdominal pain and tenderness often localised in the right lower abdomen. It often follows the onset of eosinophilic gastritis.

79 F Juvenile polyposis syndrome is a hereditary condition that is characterised by the presence of hamartomatous polyps in the digestive tract. The term juvenile polyposis refers to the type of polyp (juvenile polyp) that is found after examination of the polyp under a microscope, rather than the age at which people are diagnosed with JPS.

80 H Crohn's disease (regional enteritis) is an inflammatory disease of the intestines that may affect any part of the gastrointestinal tract from mouth to anus. It primarily causes abdominal pain, diarrhoea (which may be bloody if inflammation is at its worst), vomiting or weight loss, but may also cause complications outside the gastrointestinal tract, such as skin rashes, arthritis, inflammation of the eye, tiredness and lack of concentration. Perianal skin tags are also common in Crohn's disease.

81 G The main symptom of active ulcerative colitis is constant diarrhoea mixed with blood, of gradual onset. Sufferers also may have signs of weight loss, and blood on rectal examination. The disease is usually accompanied with different degrees of abdominal pain, from mild discomfort to severely painful cramps.

82 H OA commonly affects the hands, feet, spine and the large weight-bearing joints, such as the hips and knees. As OA progresses, the affected joints appear larger, are stiff and painful, and usually feel worse the more they are used throughout the day, thus distinguishing it from rheumatoid arthritis. In smaller joints, such as at the fingers, hard bony enlargements, called Heberden's nodes (on the distal interphalangeal joints) and/or Bouchard's nodes (on the proximal interphalangeal joints) may form.

83 F Pyrophosphate arthropathy (chondrocalcinosis) is due to the accumulation of crystals of calcium pyrophosphate dihydrate in the connective tissues. Diseases associated with chondrocalcinosis include Wilson's disease, osteoarthritis, hyperparathyroidism, haemochromatosis, hypophosphataemia and renal osteodystrophy. Radiologically, a dense line within the hyaline cartilage parallels the articular surface.

84 A Rheumatoid arthritis typically manifests with signs of inflammation, with the affected joints being swollen, warm, painful and stiff, particularly early in the morning on waking or following prolonged inactivity. Increased stiffness early in the morning is often a prominent feature of the disease and typically lasts for more than an hour.

85 E Seronegative arthritis is a classification given to the group of joint conditions with similar features to rheumatoid arthritis, but affecting different joints and lacking the specific autoantibodies used to identify rheumatoid arthritis. Rheumatoid arthritis is prevalent in the female population, whereas seronegative arthritis is more frequently seen in males. This is a case of Reiter's syndrome, which is mostly triggered by chlamydia or gastroenteritis.

86 I Pain and swelling at the first metatarsophalangeal joint should always be suspected as gout and investigated accordingly. Thiazide diuretics can trigger acute gout.

87 D An acutely inflamed, red, hot, tender swollen knee should be treated as septic until proved otherwise.

88 F Once the diagnosis of familial adenomatous polyposis is made, close colonoscopic surveillance with polypectomy is required. Prophylactic colectomy is indicated if:
- 100 polyps are present
- there are severely dysplastic polyps
- there are multiple polyps > 1 cm.

89 D Cystic fibrosis is most common among Caucasians. Ireland has both the highest incidence of cystic fibrosis in the world (almost three per 10 000), and the highest carrier rate in the world with one in 19 individuals classed as carriers.

90 C Vitamin D-resistant rickets (X-linked dominant hypophosphataemic rickets). The prevalence of the disease is 1 : 20 000. It is associated with a mutation in the *PHEX* gene sequence, located on the X chromosome.

91 J Duchenne muscular dystrophy affects one in 4000 males, making it the most prevalent of muscular dystrophies.

92 H The trigger for frontal baldness is dihydrotestosterone.

93 A Polygenic inheritance is the inheritance of quantitative traits influenced by multiple genes, such as schizophrenia.

94 J Haemorrhage typically results in reflex tachycardia prior to hypotension.

95 I The most common cause of third-degree heart block is coronary ischaemia, typically affecting the inferior region.

96 B Sinus bradycardia is common among athletes and requires no medical input.

97 C Irregular pulse should always raise suspicion of atrial fibrillation. Atrial fibrillation is more common among diabetics (by up to 40%), perhaps because they attend more regular clinical assessments, raising the possibility of early diagnosis and management, rather than any particular pathology related to diabetes. Current research may highlight an underlying possible mechanism.

98 B Femoral hernias are a relatively uncommon type, accounting for only 3% of all hernias. While femoral hernias can occur in both males and females, almost all of them develop in women because of the wider bone structure of the female pelvis.

99 C A saphena varix is a dilation of the saphenous vein at its junction with the femoral vein in the groin. It displays a cough impulse and may be mistaken for a femoral hernia. However, it has a bluish tinge and disappears on lying down. On auscultation a venous hum may be heard. It is frequently associated with varicose veins.

100 A In men, indirect hernias follow the same route as the descending testes, which migrate from the abdomen into the scrotum during the development of the urinary and reproductive organs. Men are 25 times more likely to have an inguinal hernia than women.

101 F Inguinal lymphadenopathy is typically due to an infection or malignancy.

102 H Clubbing and basal shadows point towards CFA.

103 I The clue in this question is 'shipbuilding yard', implying exposure to asbestos, resulting in mesothelioma.

104 A Bronchogenic carcinoma may be associated with paraneoplastic phenomena, e.g. Eaton–Lambert myasthaenic syndrome (muscle weakness due to autoantibodies), peripheral neuropathy, hypercalcaemia, or syndrome of inappropriate antidiuretic hormone (SIADH).

105 E Diagnosis of endocarditis is based on the clinical features and investigations such as echocardiogram, as well as any blood cultures demonstrating the presence of endocarditis-causing microorganisms.

106 B Severe diarrhoea and blood mixed with stools point to IBD.

107 G Some heart defects cause major problems immediately after birth. Others cause few, if any, problems until adulthood.

108 D Herald patch is pathognomonic of pityriasis rosea.

109 J Erythema multiforme is of unknown cause, possibly mediated by deposition of immune complex (mostly IgM) in the skin and oral mucous membrane that usually follows an infection or drug exposure. It is a common disorder, with peak incidence in the second and third decades of life. It often takes on the classical target lesion appearance. It usually resolves within 10 days.

110 B Thick-walled bullae point towards bullous pemphigoid.

111 G Thin-walled bullae point towards pemphigus vulgaris.

112 F Stevens–Johnson syndrome is a life-threatening condition affecting the skin in which cell death causes the epidermis to separate from the dermis. The syndrome is probably a hypersensitivity complex affecting the skin and the mucous membranes. Although the majority of cases are idiopathic, the main class of known causes is medications, followed by infections and cancers.

113 A In chickenpox, the blisters often appear first on the face, trunk or scalp and spread from there. Appearance of the small blisters on the scalp usually confirms the diagnosis.

114 K Koplik's spots are pathognomonic of measles. They appear on the first day of the rash. They are characterised as clustered, white lesions on the buccal mucosa near each Stenson's duct.

115 D D&Cs are commonly performed for the diagnosis of gynaecological conditions leading to abnormal uterine bleeding. As medical and non-invasive methods of abortion now exist, and because D&C requires heavy sedation or general anaesthesia and has higher risks of complication, the procedure has been declining as a method of abortion.

116 F Historically, the standard operation for the treatment of even a small invasive carcinoma of the vulva was radical vulvectomy. Surgical procedures for the treatment of carcinoma of the vulva have become more conservative and individualised to each patient. The fundamental basis of surgery for the primary tumour is now complete excision with a minimum 2-cm margin and dissection down to the deep fascia and to the periosteum of the symphysis pubis.

117 A Colporrhaphy is the surgical repair of a defect in the vaginal wall, including a cystocele (anterior) and a rectocele (posterior). An incision is made into the vaginal skin and the defect in the underlying fascia is identified. The vaginal skin is separated from the fascia and the defect is folded over and sutured. Any excess vaginal skin is removed and the incision is closed with stitches.

118 I The Manchester operation was designed for women with second- and third-degree uterine prolapse with cystourethrocele. The principle behind use of this procedure is to alter the angle of the uterus in the pelvis.

119 K Female urethral stricture disease is often treated with repeat urethral dilation or internal urethrotomy, but not always with good results. Using the vaginal wall to reconstruct large segments of the female urethra is simple and appears to have good results.

120 B Marsupialisation is the surgical technique of cutting a slit into a cyst and suturing the edges of the slit to form a continuous surface from the exterior to the interior of the cyst. Sutured in this fashion, the cyst remains open and can drain freely. This technique is used to treat a cyst when a single draining would not be effective and complete removal of the surrounding structure would not be desirable.

121 G Urethral syndrome is defined as symptoms suggestive of a lower urinary tract infection, but in the absence of significant bacteriuria with a conventional pathogen.

122 A True or total incontinence occurs when the patient has no control over the urinary flow. It is the result of communication between the ureter or bladder and the uterus or vagina.

123 C Overflow incontinence occurs when the patient's bladder is always full so that it frequently leaks urine. Weak bladder muscles, resulting in incomplete emptying of the bladder, or a blocked urethra can cause this type of incontinence.

124 F Stress incontinence is the most common form of urinary incontinence. It occurs when sudden extra pressure (stress) is placed on the bladder, resulting in urinary incontinence.

125 D Urge incontinence is involuntary loss of urine occurring for no apparent reason while feeling urinary urgency. The most common cause of urge incontinence is involuntary and inappropriate detrusor muscle contractions.

126 B UTIs are one of the most common healthcare-associated infections, accounting for 30% of all reported cases. Approximately 75% of these UTIs are associated with the use of urinary catheters.

127 G 'Snowman' sign is a rounded, figure-of-eight-like cardiac contour seen on a plain CXR of infants with total anomalous drainage of the pulmonary veins.

128 E Transposition of the great arteries is more common among babies whose mothers had gestational diabetes mellitus. D-TGA can sometimes be diagnosed in utero with an ultrasound after 18 weeks' gestation. If not, the newborn typically develops cyanosis.

129 D The boot-shaped heart sign is seen on the frontal chest radiograph of children with decreased pulmonary vasculature, as in Fallot's tetralogy.

130 C L-TGA can sometimes be diagnosed in utero with an ultrasound after 18 weeks' gestation. However, many cases of simple L-TGA are accidentally diagnosed in adulthood.

131 B In coarctation of the aorta, post-stenotic dilation of the aorta results in a classic 'figure 3' sign on X-ray.

132 I Other features of a persistent ductus arteriosus include cardiomegaly and increased pulmonary vascular markings.

133 F Callosal disorders can only be diagnosed through a brain scan. Some characteristics common in individuals with callosal disorders include vision impairments, hypotonia, poor motor coordination, delays in motor milestones such as sitting and walking, low perception of pain, delayed toilet training, and chewing and swallowing difficulties.

134 D Syringomyelia is a disorder in which a cavity forms within the spinal cord. This cavity can expand and elongate over time, destroying the spinal cord. The damage may result in pain, paralysis, weakness and stiffness in the back, shoulders and extremities.

135 G Arnold–Chiari malformation is a malformation of the brain. It consists of a downward displacement of the cerebellar tonsils through the foramen magnum. It can cause hydrocephalus, headache, fatigue, muscle weakness in the head and face, difficulty swallowing, dizziness, nausea, impaired coordination and, in severe cases, paralysis.

136 B Duchenne muscular dystrophy is a severe recessive X-linked form of muscular dystrophy characterised by rapid progression of muscle degeneration. Symptoms usually appear in male children before the age of 5.

137 J Medulloblastoma is a highly malignant primary brain tumour that originates in the cerebellum or posterior fossa. Symptoms are mainly due to secondary increased intracranial pressure due to blockage of the fourth ventricle.

138 K Tuberous sclerosis skin features include shagreen patches, skin tags, periungual fibromas, facial angiofibromas (adenoma sebaceum), hypomelanotic macules (ash leaf spots) and café au lait spots.

139 H Vasovagal syncope may present for the first time at any age. It often occurs when upright, though can occur when sitting. It rarely occurs when lying down. There are often no precipitating circumstances, but attacks are more likely to occur in certain situations, e.g. during a large meal in a warm restaurant, when watching a production in a hot theatre, when flying or after prolonged standing.

140 D Prolonged drowsiness after loss of consciousness points to epilepsy.

141 E Orthostatic hypotension (postural hypotension) is a form of hypotension in which a person's blood pressure suddenly falls when the person stands up. The decrease is typically greater than 20/10 mmHg, and may be most pronounced after resting. The incidence increases with age.

142 F Long flights can be problematic in insulin-dependent diabetic patients in view of time zone changes, which can result in inaccurate insulin doses leading to hypoglycaemia or hyperglycaemia.

143 I TIA is a change in the blood supply to a particular area of the brain, resulting in brief neurologic dysfunction that persists, by definition, for less than 24 hours. If symptoms persist longer, then it is categorised as a stroke.

144 G Stokes–Adams attack refers to a sudden, transient episode of syncope, occasionally featuring seizures. Prior to an attack, a patient may become pale, their heart rhythm experiences a temporary pause and collapse may follow. Normal periods of unconsciousness last approximately 30 seconds; if seizures are present, they will consist of twitching after 15–20 seconds. Breathing continues normally throughout the attack. Stokes–Adams attacks may be diagnosed from the history, with paleness prior to the attack and flushing after it particularly characteristic. The ECG will show asystole or ventricular fibrillation during the attacks.

145 C Anti-dsDNA shows high specificity in SLE, but a sensitivity of only 70%, which varies depending on disease activity.

146 F The most sensitive and specific antibodies for the confirmation of coeliac disease are anti-transglutaminase IgA, anti-endomysial IgA, and anti-reticulin IgA, and correlate with the degree of mucosal damage. Anti-endomysial antibody IgA can detect coeliac disease with a sensitivity and specificity of 90% and 99%.

147 K Rheumatoid factor (RF) is an IgM antibody against the Fc fragment of IgG that is present in approximately 60%–80% of patients with rheumatoid arthritis (RA). However, it is present in fewer than 40% of patients with early RA. Anti-CCP antibodies have a sensitivity and specificity equal to or better than those of rheumatoid factor, with an increased frequency of positive results in early RA. The presence of both anti-CCP antibodies and RF is highly specific for RA. Additionally, the presence of anti-CCP antibodies, like that of RF, indicates a worse prognosis.

148 A Anti-microsomal antibody (anti-thyroid peroxidase antibody) is usually positive in Hashimoto's thyroiditis. However, 10%–15% of patients with Hashimoto's thyroiditis may be antibody negative.

149 E Anti-acetylcholine receptor antibody is reliable for diagnosing autoimmune myasthenia gravis as it is positive in 74% of patients.

150 I Anti-mitochondrial antibodies can be found in 90%–95% of patients with primary biliary cirrhosis, and they have a specificity of 98% for this disease.

151 B In Wegener's granulomatosis, the most specific serologic tests are autoantibodies directed against cytoplasmic constituents of neutrophils and monocytes (c-ANCA).

152 A Bitemporal hemianopia is due to a lesion affecting the optic chiasma. It may be associated with a pituitary adenoma, craniopharyngioma, meningioma or an anterior communicating artery anuerysm.

153 D Homonymous hemianopia is usually due to a brain injury, e.g. stroke, trauma, tumours, infection or following surgery, and, rarely, it may be congenital. The pathology may involve the visual pathway anywhere from the optic tract to the visual cortex.

154 F Anton's syndrome (Anton–Babinski syndrome) is a form of cortical blindness, mostly seen following a stroke, but may also be seen after head injury. It is a form of anosognosia in which a person with partial or total blindness denies being visually impaired, despite medical evidence to the contrary. The patient typically contrives excuses for the inability to see, such as suggesting that the light is inadequate.

155 E Ipsilateral monoocular field loss is due to a lesion within the eye or the optic nerve.

156 C A lower homonymous quadrantanopia describes the loss of the same lower quadrant from each visual field. It is usually caused by damage to the optic radiation as it passes through the parietal lobe.

157 H An upper homonymous quadrantanopia describes the loss of the same upper quadrant from each visual field. It is usually caused by damage to the optic radiation as it passes through the temporal lobe.

158 E A nephrostomy is performed whenever a blockage keeps urine from passing from the kidneys, through the ureter and into the urinary bladder. Pregnancy is a relative contraindication for ESWL and PCNL.

159 B ESWL is the non-invasive treatment of kidney stones and biliary stones using an acoustic pulse. It works best with stones between 4 mm and 2 cm in diameter that are still located in the kidney. It can also be used to break up stones which are located in a ureter, but with less success.

160 C Increased urinary dilution (from forced hydration) and strong urinary alkalinisation (from oral alkalinising agents) are two of the most effective methods for the treatment and prevention of cystine kidney stones. Urinary alkalinisation works by increasing the solubility of urinary cystine.

161 F In this clinical scenario, there is a possibility that the patient may pass the stone spontaneously.

162 D Staghorn calculi refer to branched stones that fill all or part of the renal pelvis and branch into several or all of the calyces. They are most often composed of struvite (magnesium ammonium phosphate) and/or calcium carbonate apatite. These stones are often referred to as 'infection stones' since they are strongly associated with urinary tract infections with urea splitting organisms. Thus, most patients require definitive surgical treatment.

163 A Indications of PCNL include staghorn calculus (typically with ESWL), obstructive uropathy, stones in lower pole calyces and anatomical abnormalities. Contraindications for PCNL are uncorrected bleeding disorder and pregnancy (due to the risk of radiation). The other relative contraindications which may be considered are medical problems making the patient unsuitable for anaesthesia and stone location making access risky (e.g. pelvic kidney).

164 E Night blindness is one of the first signs of vitamin A deficiency. It affects vision by inhibiting the production of rhodopsin, the eye pigment responsible for sensing low light situations.

165 B Beriberi is a nervous system ailment caused by a thiamine (vitamin B_1) deficiency in the diet. The main types are wet, dry and infantile beriberi. Today, beriberi occurs mostly in patients who abuse alcohol. Drinking heavily can lead to poor nutrition, and excess alcohol makes it harder for the body to absorb and store thiamine.

166 A Scurvy is a disease resulting from a deficiency of vitamin C, which is required for the synthesis of collagen.

167 H Fibroids commonly cause menorrhagia, resulting in iron deficiency anaemia.

168 I Vitamin B_{12} (cobalamin) is absorbed at the terminal ileum.

169 G The liver uses vitamin K to synthesize blood-clotting proteins. Without vitamin K, the level of the blood-clotting proteins drops, and clotting time is prolonged.

170 J Peripheral neuropathy and CNS effects associated with the use of isoniazid are due to pyridoxine (vitamin B_6) depletion.

171 F Cough is a well-recognised side effect of ACE inhibitors.

172 D Ampicillin can trigger a significant rash if it is prescribed to a case of infectious mononucleosis (glandular fever).

173 H Myalgia is well-recognised side effect of statins, which can be checked by monitoring creatinine kinase levels.

174 I Thiazide diuretics can trigger acute gout.

175 B Neutropenia is a rare but serious side effect of carbimazole.

176 C PID is a generic term for inflammation of the uterus, fallopian tubes and/or ovaries. PID is a vague term and can refer to viral, fungal and parasitic forms, though most often caused by bacterial infections. Symptoms in PID range from asymptomatic to severe. Acute PID is highly unlikely when recent intercourse has not taken place or an IUD is not being used.

177 E Endometriosis is a gynaecological medical condition in which endometrial-like cells appear and flourish in areas outside the uterine cavity, most commonly on the ovaries. A major symptom of endometriosis is recurring pelvic pain, which is not necessarily related to the extent or stage of endometriosis. Infertility is another significant complication.

178 D In clinical practice, it is essential to exclude appendicitis and ectopic pregnancy in any young female presenting with right iliac fossa pain.

179 A Most ectopic pregnancies occur in the fallopian tube, but implantation can also occur in the cervix, ovaries and abdomen. An ectopic pregnancy is a potential medical emergency, and, if not treated properly, can lead to death.

180 J Ovarian hyperstimulation syndrome is a complication occasionally seen in women who take certain fertility medicines that stimulate egg production. The main symptoms are bloating, weight gain and abdominal pain.

181 H Septic abortion is a form of miscarriage that is associated with a serious uterine infection. Infection may spread to other parts of the body and cause septicaemia.

182 D In cervical carcinoma, stage II refers to invasion beyond cervix, stage IIA, without parametrial invasion, but involving the upper two-thirds of the vagina, and stage IIB, with parametrial invasion.

183 A Endometrial carcinoma is surgically staged using the FIGO cancer staging system. Stage IIA implies endocervical glandular involvement only. In 2010, the FIGO staging system was modified and stage II implies cervical stromal invasion, but not beyond the uterus.

184 H In cervical carcinoma, stage III refers to the extension to the pelvic wall or lower third of the vagina, stage IIIA involves the lower third of the vagina, and stage IIIB extends to the pelvic wall and/or causes hydronephrosis or non-functioning kidney.

185 K In ovarian carcinoma, stage IIA refers to involvement of one or both ovaries, with extension or implants onto the uterus or fallopian tube, and negative peritoneal washings.

186 C In endometrial carcinoma, stage IIIA (FIGO staging system) means that the tumour invaded the serosa or adnexa, or positive malignant peritoneal cytology.

187 I Vaginal carcinoma stage III means that cancer has spread outside the vagina and reached the side walls of the pelvis with or without lymphadenopathy.

188 F Digital clubbing is not an accurate gauge of the severity of lung damage in cystic fibrosis patients. The extent of the clubbing is different for almost every individual, and doesn't progress as the disease progresses. There is no way to treat or reverse digital clubbing, but it is also a benign symptom.

189 H Laryngomalacia is a very common condition of infancy in which the soft immature cartilage of the upper larynx collapses inward during inhalation, causing airway obstruction. The noise is more pronounced when the patient is on his or her back (with gravity making the epiglottis fall backwards).

190 A Pulmonary sequestration is a cystic or solid mass composed of non-functioning primitive tissue that does not communicate with the tracheobronchial tree and has anomalous systemic blood supply. The two forms of pulmonary sequestration are intrapulmonary, which is surrounded by normal lung tissue, and extrapulmonary, which has its own pleural investment.

191 G Most patients with pulmonary arteriovenous malformations have the autosomal dominant disease hereditary haemorrhagic telangiectasia. Symptoms caused by pulmonary arteriovenous malformations are often insidious, as the arteriovenous malformations slowly enlarge. Dyspnoea, especially with exercise, may develop over many years. Haemoptysis and, rarely, massive haemoptysis may occur. Less common complaints include chest pain and cough.

192 J TEFs are a common congenital anomaly with an incidence of one case in 3000 live births. Acquired TEFs are quite rare.

193 B Signs which occur during an asthma attack include the use of accessory muscles of respiration, tachypnoea, tachycardia, paradoxical pulse (a pulse that is weaker during inhalation and stronger during exhalation), hyperexpansion of the chest and cyanosis.

194 G Analysis of the pleural fluid is the single best method to determine the cause of a pleural effusion. Thoracentesis should be performed when sufficient fluid is present to allow a safe procedure, except when the suspected effusion is clearly secondary to a specific underlying disease. Ultrasonography in experienced hands is superior to CXR for detecting pleural effusion. Ultrasonography can easily distinguish between free and loculated pleural effusion and allow differentiation of pleural fluid from pleural thickening and solid masses.

195 C Chest radiography leads to the diagnosis of tracheo-oesophageal fistula in most cases, and other investigations are rarely required.

196 C While peak expiratory flow rates provide a useful first line assessment, a CXR may be necessary to exclude other causes of persistent cough.

197 E In trauma, where it may not be possible to perform an upright film, chest radiography may miss up to a third of pneumothoraces, while CT remains very sensitive. It is also useful in identifying underlying lung pathology in pneumothorax.

198 B Despite advances in non-invasive diagnostic techniques, contrast-enhanced pulmonary angiography remains the criterion standard in the diagnosis of pulmonary arteriovenous malformations.

199 F Laryngoscopy offers the best means to confirm the diagnosis. However, in an infant with typical inspiratory noises (worse when supine) who have a normal cry and normal growth and development, clinical diagnosis is not unreasonable.

200 A The most serious potential adverse effect of metformin is lactic acidosis. When there is impaired renal function, clearance of metformin and lactate is reduced, leading to increased levels of both and possibly causing lactic acidosis. Accordingly, metformin dose should be reduced in diabetic patients with an eGFR of 60–90 ml/min. It should not be used when the eGFR is < 30 ml/min.

201 I Phenytoin toxicity may also cause hallucinations, confusion and diplopia.

202 D Bleomycin is a recognised cause of lung fibrosis.

203 E Amiodarone side effects feature frequently in PLAB tests as it is commonly used in the management of arrhythmias.

204 H Lithium may cause nephrogenic diabetes insipidus, hypothyroidism and nystagmus.

205 B *Clostridium difficile* is the most serious cause of antibiotic-associated diarrhoea. Mild cases of *C. difficile* infection can be cured simply by discontinuing the antibiotics responsible. In more serious cases, oral metronidazole or vancomycin are the treatments of choice.

206 E PBC is an autoimmune disease of the liver marked by the slow progressive destruction of bile canaliculi resulting in cholestasis, which then leads to scarring, fibrosis and cirrhosis. The sex ratio is at least 9 : 1 (female to male). Anti-nuclear antibodies appear to be prognostic agents in PBC. Anti-glycoprotein-210 antibodies and anti-P62 antibodies correlate with progression towards end-stage liver failure. Anti-centromere antibodies correlate with developing portal hypertension.

207 B Chronic active hepatitis, is a syndrome with a varied aetiology, but similar histological appearances on liver biopsy. There is chronic hepatic necrosis and fibrosis which in most cases progresses to cirrhosis and liver failure. It may be autoimmune, viral, metabolic (Wilson's disease, haemochromatosis or alcohol), drug-induced or due to alpha-1-antitrypsin deficiency.

208 J Hepatic adenomas are often seen in young women who use oral contraceptives. The lesions can occasionally regress after cessation of oral contraceptives. Rarely, hepatic adenomas may undergo malignant transformation to hepatocellular carcinoma.

209 G Wilson's disease (hepatolenticular degeneration) is an autosomal recessive disorder in which copper accumulates in tissues. This manifests as neurological, psychiatric symptoms and/or liver disease. There is no totally reliable test for Wilson's disease, but levels of ceruloplasmin and copper in the blood, as well of the amount of copper excreted in urine during a 24-hour period, are useful to reach a diagnosis. The gold standard is a liver biopsy. Penicillamine is usually the first treatment used.

210 C Gaucher's disease is a genetic disease caused by a recessive mutation in a gene located on chromosome 1, resulting in deficiency of glucocerebrosidase. The carrier rate among Ashkenazi Jews is about 9%.

211 A Gilbert's syndrome is the most common hereditary cause of increased bilirubin and is found in 5%–10% of the population. It has an autosomal recessive inheritance pattern. It is characterised by jaundice, caused by elevated levels of serum unconjugated bilirubin.

212 H 'The Pill' is one of the most commonly used treatments for endometriosis, and is a good choice for young women with mild disease who also require effective contraception.

213 C This is a young patient with a mild disease and a relatively short history of infertility, so it would be wise to wait.

214 E Conservative therapy consists of the excision (cystectomy) of the endometrium, adhesions, resection of endometriomas and restoration of normal pelvic anatomy as much as possible.

215 B Radical therapy in endometriosis includes hysterectomy and bilateral salpingo-oophorectomy. Radical surgery is generally reserved for women with chronic pelvic pain that is disabling and treatment resistant. As this patient is premenopausal, she would be a candidate for oestrogen replacement therapy.

216 G Progesterone has proven efficacy in pain suppression. It counteracts oestrogen and inhibits the growth of the endometrium. Such therapy can reduce or eliminate menstruation in a controlled and reversible fashion.

217 H Combined oral contraceptive pill is a useful treatment for primary dysmenorrhoea.

218 C Hypothyroidism in its early stages may be associated with hyperprolactinaemia.

219 A The long duration of amenorrhoea with lack of any symptoms suggestive of pregnancy or hypothyroidism makes pregnancy or hypothyroidism unlikely. In this case, it is essential to check prolactin levels, as slightly elevated prolactin levels may not necessarily result in galactorrhoea, but could result in reduction in menstrual flow or amenorrhoea.

220 D Sheehan's syndrome (post-partum hypopituitarism) is caused by pituitary necrosis due to blood loss and hypovolaemic shock during and after childbirth.

221 E Turner's syndrome may be diagnosed by amniocentesis during pregnancy. Karyotyping is the test of choice to diagnose Turner's syndrome.

222 K Ectopic pregnancy needs to be excluded in view of the amenorrhoea and right-side tenderness with normal uterine size. A pelvic ultrasound scan is the investigation of choice here. Repeating the β-HCG levels is the second-best option (expecting it to drop or slightly increase).

223 G CA 19-9 is elevated in patients with pancreatic cancer or colonic cancer.

224 E CA 125 is the most commonly used marker for ovarian cancer. CEA is elevated in patients with colorectal carcinoma, gastric carcinoma, pancreatic carcinoma, lung carcinoma and breast carcinoma, as well as medullary thyroid carcinoma.

225 C CA 15-3 (carcinoma antigen 15-3) is a tumour marker for breast cancer.

226 H Prostatic cancer is monitored by PSA.

227 J Raised AFP may be seen in testicular cancer, ovarian cancer, hepatoma, stomach cancer or pancreatic cancer.

228 D Radioiodine therapy is not used at any time in pregnant women because of the risk of foetal hypothyroidism. Accordingly, antithyroid drugs (specifically carbimazole and propylthiouracil in the UK) are used. However, there are two concerns about antithyroid drugs for thyrotoxicosis: that the drugs cause hypothyroidism in the foetus and that they have teratogenic effects. Doses of antithyroid drugs should be maintained at the lowest dose needed to keep the mother's FT4 level in the high–normal range.

229 D Antithyroid drugs are prescribed either for the short-term control of thyrotoxicosis prior to definitive treatment, or in the hope of achieving remission in patients with Graves' disease, especially in those presenting under the age of 40. Generally, a course of

18 months is recommended, but the probability of achieving long-term remission is less than 50%. The significance of keloid scar is that it makes surgery a less attractive option.

230 B While thyroidectomy is no longer the recommended first-line therapy for hyperthyroid Graves' disease, it may be appropriate in the presence of a thyroid nodule that is suggestive of carcinoma or in patients with large goitres.

231 B The outcome of subtotal thyroidectomy is usually excellent. However, most patients will need to take thyroid hormone replacement for the rest of their lives.

232 F Hashimoto's thyroiditis (chronic lymphocytic thyroiditis) is an autoimmune disease in which the thyroid gland is gradually destroyed by a variety of cell- and antibody-mediated immune processes. It often results in hypothyroidism with episodes of hyperthyroidism. Hypothyroidism caused by Hashimoto's thyroiditis is treated with thyroxine.

233 A Varicella pneumonia can range from mild to severe, and the prognosis depends upon severity and treatment. If the illness is contracted by someone with neoplastic disease, the prognosis is poor. If the person is pregnant, an acyclovir regimen is recommended. The use of corticosteroids is controversial because it can cause rapid improvement in some cases, but has also proved to be completely ineffective in others.

234 E The diagnosis of bronchiectasis is based on the review of clinical history and characteristic patterns in high-resolution CT scan findings. It is important to appreciate that chest radiographs may be negative in patients with minor to moderate disease.

235 I Kerley lines are a sign seen on chest radiographs with interstitial pulmonary oedema. They are thin linear pulmonary opacities caused by fluid or cellular infiltration into the interstitium of the lungs. They are suggestive for the diagnosis of congestive heart failure, but are also seen in various non-cardiac conditions, such as pulmonary fibrosis, interstitial deposition of heavy metal particles or carcinomatosis of the lung.

236 C Those are classic features of lobar consolidation.

237 B In clinical practice, we rarely come across such features nowadays, as such patients are usually diagnosed and treated before progressing to that stage. In addition, it is much easier and more reliable to diagnose valvular lesions via an echocardiogram.

238 F Those radiological findings reflect the complications of ASD.

239 J Both NSAIDs and steroids can cause significant gastritis and gastric bleeding. It is important to prescribe a PPI for such patients for gastric protection.

240 H Macrocytic anaemia can be classified as megaloblastic and non-megaloblastic. Megaloblastic refers to a characteristic abnormality of the erythroblasts in the bone marrow in which the maturation of the nucleus is delayed relative to the cytoplasm. It results from defective DNA synthesis. Megaloblastic anaemia is usually due to vitamin B_{12} or folic acid deficiency. Non-megaloblastic anaemia is due to alcoholism, hypothyroidism and liver disease. In addition, alcoholism results in several vitamin deficiencies due to malnutrition and the toxic effect of alcohol, which may also explain why macrocytic anaemia is common in alcoholics.

241 A Pernicious anaemia is a type of megaloblastic anaemia. It is caused by loss of gastric parietal cells and subsequent inability to absorb vitamin B_{12}. A greater association than anticipated exists between pernicious anaemia and other autoimmune diseases, which include thyroid disorders, type 1 diabetes mellitus, ulcerative colitis and Addison's disease.

242 I PNH is a rare, acquired, potentially life-threatening disease of the blood characterised by complement-induced intravascular haemolytic anaemia, red urine (due to the appearance of haemoglobin in the urine) and thrombosis.

243 G The occurrence of AIHA in patients with non-Hodgkin's lymphoma is well known.

244 B Acute haemolysis in people with G6PD deficiency can be triggered by antimalarial drugs, e.g. primaquine, pamaquine and chloroquine. There is evidence that other antimalarials may also exacerbate G6PD deficiency, but only at higher doses. Sulfonamides and aspirin should also be avoided by people with G6PD deficiency, as should certain analgesics and a few non-sulfa antibiotics, e.g. nalidixic acid, nitrofurantoin, isoniazid and ciprofloxacin.

245 D Those are classic features of iron deficiency anaemia.

246 A α-thalassaemias involve the genes *HBA1* and *HBA2*, inherited in a Mendelian recessive fashion. There are two gene loci and so four alleles. It is also connected to the deletion of the 16p chromosome. α-thalassaemias result in decreased α-globin production, resulting in an excess of β-chains in adults and excess γ-chains in newborns.

247 I Those are classic features of anaemia of chronic disease, which is more common in the elderly.

248 J Spherocytosis is caused by a molecular defect in one or more of the proteins of the red blood cell cytoskeleton, including spectrin and ankyrin. Because the cell skeleton has a defect, the blood cell contracts to its most surface-tension efficient and least flexible configuration, a sphere.

249 C In PNH, red blood cells are destroyed as they lack the proteins that protect them from complement, resulting in anaemia. The increased rate of thrombosis is due to dysfunction of platelets due to binding by complement, or possibly due to low nitric oxide levels.

250 B Von Willebrand disease is the most common hereditary coagulation abnormality, although it can also be acquired as a result of other medical conditions. It arises from a qualitative or quantitative deficiency of Von Willebrand factor.

251 A Wilms' tumour (nephroblastoma) is cancer of the kidneys that typically occurs in children. Most nephroblastomas are unilateral, being bilateral in less than 5% of cases.

252 B Non-Hodgkin's lymphomas are a diverse group of cancers that include any kind of lymphoma except Hodgkin's lymphomas. They vary significantly in their severity, from indolent to very aggressive. The left supraclavicular mass refers to Virchow's node, which is typically enlarged (Troisier's sign) in gastrointestinal malignancies, and also in lymphomas.

253 I Lymphadenitis typically causes pain, tenderness, and lymph node enlargement. Pain and tenderness typically distinguish lymphadenitis from lymphadenopathy. With some infections, the overlying skin is inflamed, occasionally with cellulitis. Abscesses may form, and penetration to the skin produces draining sinuses. Fever is common. The underlying cause is usually suggested by history and examination. If not, aspiration and culture or excisional biopsy is indicated.

254 G Neuroblastoma is the most common extracranial solid cancer in childhood and the most common cancer in infancy. Neuroblastoma often spreads to other parts of the body before any symptoms are apparent and 50%–60% of all neuroblastoma cases present with metastases. The first symptoms of neuroblastoma are often vague, making diagnosis difficult. Fatigue, loss of appetite, fever and joint pain are common. Symptoms depend on primary tumour locations and metastases if present.

255 E Medulloblastoma is a highly malignant primary brain tumour that originates in the cerebellum or posterior fossa. Symptoms are mainly due to secondary increased intracranial pressure due to blockage of the fourth ventricle and are usually present for up to 5 months before diagnosis is made.

256 D Ewing's sarcoma is a malignant round-cell tumour. It is a rare disease in which cancer cells are found in the bone or in soft tissue. The most common areas in which it occurs are the pelvis, the femur, the humerus, the ribs and clavicle. Ewing's sarcoma occurs most frequently in male teenagers.

257 B Type 1 second-degree AV block, also known as Mobitz I or Wenckebach, is almost always a disease of the AV node. This is almost always a benign condition for which no specific treatment is needed. Most people with Wenckebach do not show symptoms.

258 K Type 2 second-degree AV block, also known as Mobitz II, is almost always a disease of the distal conduction system (His–Purkinje system). The medical significance of this type of AV block is that it may progress rapidly to complete heart block.

259 E Sinus arrhythmia is a naturally occurring variation in heart rate that occurs during a breathing cycle.

260 H WPW is a syndrome of pre-excitation of ventricles of the heart due to an accessory pathway known as the bundle of Kent. This accessory pathway is an abnormal electrical communication from the atria to the ventricles. WPW is a type of atrioventricular reentrant tachycardia. Its incidence is about 0.2% among the population. While the vast majority of individuals with a bundle of Kent remain asymptomatic throughout their entire lives, there is a risk of sudden death associated with the syndrome. An ECG will show the characteristic delta wave.

261 D An ECG is routinely done on patients with chest pain to quickly diagnose myocardial infarctions. An ECG may show signs of right heart strain or acute cor pulmonale in cases of large pulmonary emboli. The most commonly seen signs in the ECG are sinus tachycardia, right axis deviation and right bundle branch block.

262 A RBBB is mostly asymptomatic. Prevalence of RBBB increases with age. A mnemonic to remember the ECG changes is WiLLiaM MaRRoW, i.e. with LBBB there is a W in V_1 and an M in V_6, and with an RBBB there is an M in lead V_1 and a W in lead V_6.

263 F Anxiety neurosis is the most common form of psychoneurosis occurring among individuals of above average intelligence.

264 A Depression is quite common and about one in 10 people will experience depression at some point. It is very different from the common experience of feeling unhappy, miserable or fed up for a short period of time. Women are more likely to have depression than men. Depression can affect people of any age, including children.

265 J Somatisation disorder is a psychiatric diagnosis applied to patients who persistently complain of varied physical symptoms that have no identifiable physical origin. The disorder may begin before 30 years of age and could last for several years, resulting in either medical-seeking behaviour or significant treatment.

266 G Mania is a state of abnormally elevated or irritable mood, arousal and/or energy levels. Mania varies in intensity, from mild mania (hypomania) to full-blown mania with psychotic features including hallucinations, delusions of grandeur, paranoia, catatonic behaviour, aggression and self-neglect.

267 C Schizophrenia is a mental disorder characterised by the disintegration of thought processes and emotional responsiveness. It most commonly manifests as auditory hallucinations, paranoid or bizarre delusions, or disorganised speech and thinking, and is accompanied by significant social and occupational dysfunction. The mainstay of treatment is antipsychotic medication, which primarily works by suppressing dopamine activity. Psychotherapy and vocational and social rehabilitation are also important.

268 H OCD is an anxiety disorder characterised by intrusive thoughts that produce uneasiness, apprehension, fear or worry, and by repetitive behaviours aimed at reducing anxiety, or by a combination of such obsessions and behaviours.

269 E Phaeochromocytoma is a neuroendocrine tumour of the medulla of the adrenal glands (originating in the chromaffin cells), or extra-adrenal chromaffin tissue that failed to involute after birth and secretes excessive amounts of catecholamines (usually adrenaline if in the adrenal gland and not extra-adrenal), and noradrenaline. The signs and symptoms of a phaeochromocytoma are those of sympathetic nervous system hyperactivity.

270 B MEN type 1 is an inherited disorder in which persons develop tumours of the parathyroid glands, the enteropancreatic neuroendocrine system, the anterior pituitary gland and the skin. The most common endocrine tumours are parathyroid tumours that cause hyperparathyroidism and hypercalcaemia. Other tumours include gastrinomas, insulinomas, prolactinomas and carcinoid tumours. MEN 1 is caused by a defect in a gene that carries the code for a protein called menin.

271 D Carcinoid syndrome refers to a group of symptoms that occur secondary to carcinoid tumours. The syndrome includes flushing (the most important clinical finding, usually of the head and the upper part of thorax) and diarrhoea, and, less frequently, heart failure and bronchoconstriction. It is caused by endogenous secretion of mainly serotonin and kallikrein. It occurs in approximately 10% of carcinoid tumours.

272 C MEN type 2 is a rare familial cancer syndrome caused by mutations in the RET proto-oncogene. Inherited as an autosomal dominant disorder, MEN 2 has three distinct subtypes: MEN 2A, MEN 2B and familial medullary thyroid carcinoma. Medullary thyroid carcinoma (MTC) represents the most frequent initial diagnosis. Occasionally, phaeochromocytoma and primary hyperparathyroidism may be the initial diagnosis.

MEN 2A associates medullary thyroid carcinoma with phaeochromocytoma in about 20%–50% of cases, and with primary hyperparathyroidism in 5%–20% of cases. MEN 2B associates medullary thyroid carcinoma with phaeochromocytoma in 50% of cases, with marfanoid habitus and with mucosal and digestive ganglioneuromatosis.

273 A Parathyroid adenomas can be due to a genetic problem. The most common cause of parathyroid adenoma is hyperparathyroidism. Women over 60 have the highest risk for developing this condition. Radiation to the head or neck also increases the risk.

274 G In Gilbert's syndrome, the cause of hyperbilirubinaemia is the reduced activity of glucuronyltransferase, which conjugates bilirubin. Conjugation renders the bilirubin water-soluble, after which it is excreted in bile into the duodenum.

275 D PSC is a chronic liver disease caused by progressive inflammation and scarring of the bile ducts of the liver. The cause of PSC is unknown, although it is thought to be an autoimmune disorder. There is an increased prevalence of HLA alleles A1, B8 and DR3 in primary sclerosing cholangitis.

276 L Jaundice presenting after cholecystectomy may be the initial manifestation of a serious surgical complication and requires rigorous diagnostic pursuit and therapeutic intervention. Biloma is a well recognised post-cholecystectomy complication that often accompanies biliary ductal injury. Dropped calculus post-laparoscopic cholecystectomy is another complication, but it is usually painful. Fever may be associated with an infected biloma or cholangitis.

277 C The initial presentation of pancreatic cancer varies according to its location. Malignancies in the pancreatic body or tail usually present with pain and weight loss, while those in the head of the pancreas typically present with steatorrhea, weight loss and jaundice. The recent onset of atypical diabetes mellitus, thrombophlebitis (Trousseau's sign), or pancreatitis are sometimes noted. Courvoisier's sign defines the presence of jaundice and a painlessly distended gall bladder as strongly indicative of pancreatic cancer, and may be used to distinguish pancreatic cancer from gallstones.

278 A Sjögren's syndrome is closely linked to primary biliary cirrhosis.

279 C Numbness and tingling in the fingers is due to carpal tunnel syndrome, which may be associated with hypothyroidism (due to fluid retention). Deafness is also another feature of hypothyroidism.

280 G Meningitis caused by *Neisseria meningitidis* can be differentiated from meningitis due to other causes by a rapidly spreading petechial rash which may precede other symptoms. The rash consists of numerous petechiae on the trunk, lower limbs, mucous membranes, conjuctiva and the palms of the hands or soles of the feet. The rash is typically non-blanching: the redness does not disappear when pressed with a finger or a glass tumbler (glass test). Although this rash is not necessarily present in meningococcal meningitis, it is relatively specific for the disease.

281 J Small cell (oat cell) carcinoma of bronchus may be associated with inappropriate antidiuretic hormone secretion (SIADH) resulting in hyponatraemia.

282 B LSD is an ergoline derivative. It is commonly synthesised by reacting diethylamine with an activated form of lysergic acid. LSD stimulates centres of the sympathetic nervous system in the midbrain, which leads to pupillary dilation, increase in body temperature and rise in the blood-sugar level. LSD also has a serotonin-blocking effect. It should be noted that there is no 'safe dose' for LSD, so the term 'LSD overdose' is rather inaccurate.

283 I Hypoglycaemia due to excessive insulin is the most common type of serious hypoglycaemia. Mild cases can be managed by eating or drinking 10–30 g of carbohydrates. When hypoglycaemia is more severe or carbohydrates cannot be given by mouth, glucagon can be injected intramuscularly or intravenously, or dextrose can be infused intravenously to raise the blood glucose.

284 D Falls among the elderly are rather common and it is crucial to obtain a very detailed history. Focus should be directed towards possible causes, e.g. postural hypotension, cardiac arrhythmia, vasovagal syncope or epilepsy, as well as possible complications, e.g. subdural haematoma. In this case, biting of the tongue as well as incontinence, point towards epilepsy.

285 B Those are classic features of aspirin overdose.

286 E The majority of the TCAs act primarily as serotonin-norepinephrine reuptake inhibitors (SNRIs) by blocking the serotonin transporter (SERT) and the norepinephrine transporter (NET), respectively, which results in an elevation of the extracellular concentrations of these neurotransmitters, and therefore an enhancement of neurotransmission. The TCAs also have varying but typically high affinity for antagonising the H_1 and H_2 histamine receptors, as well as the muscarinic acetylcholine receptors. As a result, they also act as potent antihistamines and anticholinergics. That explains the clinical features of TCA overdose.

287 G Those are classic features of β-blocker overdose.

288 K Digoxin toxicity is characterised by many features, specifically disturbances of colour vision with a tendency to yellow-green colouring, nausea, vomiting, anorexia and diarrhoea. ECG changes include ST depression and T wave inversion in V_5–V_6 in a reversed tick pattern, bradycardia, prolonged PR, shortened QT and arrhythmias, especially heart block or bigeminy.

289 A The toxic syndrome occurs at levels above 1.4 mmol/L and involves a decreased appetite, diarrhoea, vomiting, ataxia, nystagmus, dysarthria, confusion and epileptic seizures. Toxicity may lead to coma with hyperreflexia and increased muscle tone. A few patients may sustain irreversible neurological damage. Significant lithium toxicity may occur when lithium is allowed to interact with sodium-depleting drugs, especially diuretics.

290 H Paracetamol overdose is very common in the UK. It is the most common cause of acute liver failure. Commonly, patients are asymptomatic for the first 24 hours or have non-specific abdominal symptoms. Hepatic necrosis begins to develop after 24 hours (elevated transaminases, RUQ pain and jaundice) and can progress to acute liver failure.

291 H Bronchiectasis is characterised by localised, irreversible dilation of part of the bronchial tree caused by destruction of the muscle and elastic tissue. Involved bronchi are dilated, inflamed and easily collapsible, resulting in airflow obstruction and impaired clearance of secretions. Bronchiectasis is associated with a wide range of disorders, but it usually results from necrotising bacterial infections, such as infections caused by *Staphylococci*, *Klebsiella* or *Bordetella pertussis*. It is classified as an obstructive lung disease, along with emphysema, bronchitis and cystic fibrosis.

292 A One of the serious complications of a total hip replacement is deep venous thrombosis which may then result in pulmonary embolism.

293 G Pneumonia is common, occurring in all age groups and is a leading cause of death among the young, the old and the chronically ill.

294 J Wegener's granulomatosis is a form of vasculitis affecting the lungs, kidneys and other organs. Rhinitis is generally the first sign in most patients; saddle-nose deformity due to a perforated septum is rather characteristic. Cytoplasmic staining ANCAs that react with the enzyme proteinase 3 (cANCA) in neutrophils are associated with Wegener's.

295 F The main types of lung cancer are small cell lung carcinoma and non-small cell lung carcinoma. This distinction is important, because the treatment varies: non-small cell lung carcinoma is sometimes treated with surgery, while small cell lung carcinoma usually responds better to chemotherapy and radiation. The most common cause of lung cancer is smoking.

296 B Classic symptoms of TB are a chronic cough with bloodstained sputum, fever, night sweats and weight loss. Transmission can only occur from people with active, not latent, TB.

297 K *HLA*-B27 is associated with ankylosing spondylitis, Reiter's syndrome, acute anterior uveitis and iritis, psoriatic arthritis and ulcerative colitis-associated spondyloarthritis.

298 D *HLA*-DR3 is associated with primary Sjögren's syndrome, autoimmune hepatitis and type 1 diabetes mellitus.

299 A *HLA*-DR7 is associated with psoriasis vulgaris and coeliac disease.

300 G *HLA*-DR4 is associated with type 1 diabetes mellitus and rheumatoid arthritis.

301 I *HLA*-A3 is associated with myasthenia gravis.

302 F *HLA*-DQ8 is associated with papillary thyroid carcinomas, early onset pauciarticular juvenile chronic arthritis and primary biliary cirrhosis.

303 D Congenital adrenal hyperplasia refers to any of several autosomal recessive diseases resulting from mutations of genes for enzymes mediating the biochemical steps of production of cortisol from cholesterol by the adrenal glands. It is one of the possible underlying synthesis problems in Addison's disease. Depending on clinical features, treatment may include glucocorticoids, mineralocorticoids, androgens and/or oestrogens.

304 C Primary dysmenorrhoea is caused by the release of prostaglandins and other inflammatory mediators in the uterus resulting in painful uterine contractions.

305 A Dysfunctional uterine bleeding is found in the absence of demonstrable structural or organic pathology. Diagnosis is made by exclusion, as organic pathology must first be ruled out. Ten per cent of cases occur in women who are ovulating, while 90% occur in women who are not ovulating. Mid-cycle oestrogen and late-cycle progestin can be used for mid- and late-cycle bleeding, respectively.

306 F Isosexual precocious puberty refers to the appearance of phenotypically appropriate secondary sexual characteristics before age 8 years in girls and before 9 years in boys.

307 H Clomiphene is a selective oestrogen receptor modulator (SERM) that increases production of gonadotropins by inhibiting negative feedback on the hypothalamus. It is used mainly for ovarian stimulation in female infertility due to anovulation.

308 E Choriocarcinoma is a malignant, trophoblastic and aggressive cancer, usually of the placenta. It is characterised by early blood spread to the lungs. Choriocarcinoma is one of the tumours that are most sensitive to chemotherapy. The cure rate, even for metastatic choriocarcinoma, is around 90%–95%. Virtually everyone without metastases can be cured. At present, treatment with methotrexate or actinomycin D is recommended for low-risk disease.

309 E Early symptoms of ectopic pregnancy are either absent or subtle. Clinical presentation occurs at a range of 5–8 weeks. Vaginal bleeding is usually mild as an ectopic pregnancy is usually a failing pregnancy and falling levels of progesterone from the corpus luteum on the ovary cause withdrawal bleeding.

310 B Molar pregnancy is an abnormal form of pregnancy, wherein a non-viable, fertilised egg implants in the uterus and thereby converts normal pregnancy processes into pathological ones. The placenta contains grape-like vesicles that are usually visible with the naked eye. The vesicles arise by distention of the chorionic villi by fluid.

311 C Any vaginal bleeding other than spotting during early pregnancy is considered a threatened miscarriage. About one in every four pregnant women has some bleeding during the first few months. About half of these women stop bleeding and have a normal pregnancy. The bleeding and pain associated with threatened miscarriage are usually mild.

312 D Physiological amenorrhoea occurs before puberty, during pregnancy and lactation, or during and after menopause.

313 H Hypogonadotrophic amenorrhoea means there is a problem in the hypothalamus or pituitary gland. This type of amenorrhoea is associated with low levels of sex hormones (FSH, LH and GnRH).

314 I Eugonadotrophic amenorrhoea is associated with congenital abnormalities of the genital tract.

315 E Post-operative shortness of breath and chest pain should always be investigated to exclude pulmonary embolism.

316 A Most patients with aortic dissection present with severe pain that had a sudden onset. The location of pain is associated with the location of the dissection. Anterior chest pain is associated with ascending aorta dissections, while interscapular pain is associated with descending aortic dissections. While the pain may be confused with the pain of a myocardial infarction, aortic dissection is usually not associated with the other signs that suggest myocardial infarction, including heart failure, and ECG changes. Also, individuals suffering from an aortic dissection usually do not present with profuse sweating.

317 I Raised JVP and ankle oedema points to right ventricular failure. In this case, it is most probably secondary to acute right ventricular infarction, in view of the epigastric chest pain.

318 C Boerhaave's syndrome is rupture of the oesophageal wall due to vomiting. The most common anatomical location of the tear in Boerhaave's syndrome is the left posterolateral wall of the lower third of the oesophagus, 2–3 cm before the stomach. Within a few hours to days, pleural effusion with or without pneumothorax, widened mediastinum and subcutaneous emphysema are typically seen.

319 G HCM is frequently asymptomatic until sudden cardiac death, and is the leading cause of sudden cardiac death in young athletes. History and physical examination alone are ineffective, giving warning of heart abnormalities in only 3% of patients before sudden cardiac death. HCM can be detected with an echocardiogram with an accuracy > 80%. Treatment of symptoms of obstructive HCM is directed towards decreasing the left ventricular outflow tract gradient and symptoms of dyspnoea, chest pain and syncope. The first medication that is routinely used is a β-blocker. If symptoms and gradient persist, disopyramide may be added. Alternately, a calcium channel blocker such as verapamil may be substituted for a β-blocker.

320 F Kawasaki disease is an autoimmune disease that manifests as a systemic necrotising medium-sized vessel vasculitis and is largely seen in children under 5 years of age. It affects many organ systems, mainly those including the blood vessels, skin, mucous membranes and lymph nodes; however, its most serious effect is on the heart, where it can cause severe coronary artery aneurysms in untreated children. Aspirin remains an important part of the treatment but salicylates alone are not as effective as IV immunoglobulins.

321 A TIA is due to a reduction in the blood supply to a particular area of the brain, resulting in brief neurologic deficit that persists, by definition, for less than 24 hours. If symptoms persist longer, then it is categorised as a stroke. A cerebral infarct that lasts longer than 24 hours but less than 72 hours is termed a reversible ischaemic neurologic deficit (RIND). The most common cause of a TIA is an embolus dislodged from an atherosclerotic plaque in one of the carotid arteries or from a thrombus because of atrial fibrillation.

322 K The incidence of VBI increases with age and typically occurs in the seventh or eighth decade of life. Reflecting atherosclerosis, which is the most common cause of VBI, it affects men twice as often as women. VBI occurs when the neck is overextended, damaging the blood vessels in the neck and disrupting the blood flow to the brain, resulting in a potential stroke. The vertigo due to VBI may be reproduced by head turning, which could occlude the ipsilateral vertebral artery and result in decreased blood flow to the brain if the contralateral artery is occluded.

323 D Lateral medullary syndrome (Wallenberg syndrome) is caused by posterior inferior cerebellar artery syndrome insufficiency. It is characterised by a loss of pain and temperature sensation on the contralateral side of the body and ipsilateral side of the face. This crossed finding is diagnostic for the syndrome. Clinical symptoms include dysphagia, slurred speech, ataxia, facial pain, vertigo, nystagmus, diplopia and Horner's syndrome.

324 E Symptoms of SAH include a sudden severe headache, vomiting, confusion, and occasionally seizures. The diagnosis is usually confirmed with a head CT scan. In 85% of cases of spontaneous SAH, the cause is rupture of a cerebral aneurysm in the circle of Willis and its branches.

325 F Subdural haematomas are most often caused by head injury, when rapidly changing velocities within the skull may stretch and tear small bridging veins that cross the subdural space. Subdural haematomas are divided into acute, subacute and chronic, depending on their speed of onset.

326 B Percutaneous transluminal angioplasty of the femoral artery is one method that has been used for many years, especially for patients with a high level of surgical risk. The use of stents alongside the traditional balloon techniques has further improved the results.

327 C Femoro-distal bypass is performed either using a long vein from the leg or using a synthetic graft. Incisions are made in the groin of the affected leg, inside the thigh region and in the calf, ankle or foot. The graft is joined from the femoral artery in the upper leg to one of the arteries in the lower calf below the knee by means of a tunnel through the muscle layer or under the skin.

328 D Tissue plasminogen activator is a protein involved in the breakdown of blood clots. It may be manufactured using recombinant biotechnology techniques, known as recombinant tissue plasminogen activator (rtPA), e.g. alteplase and reteplase.

329 A Femoro-popliteal bypass surgery is used to bypass diseased blood vessels above or below the knee. A newer, minimally-invasive procedure is percutaneous transluminal angioplasty (PTA) of the femoral arteries.

330 F Fasciotomy is a surgical procedure where the fascia is cut to relieve tension or pressure, thus restoring circulation to an area of tissue or muscle. Fasciotomy is a limb-saving procedure when used to treat acute compartment syndrome.

331 B Follicular adenoma of the thyroid is a common benign tumour of the thyroid gland. They present as a solitary nodule, usually as a painless mass. Follicular adenomas can be described as 'cold', 'warm' or 'hot', depending on their level of function. Hyperthyroidism of toxic adenomas generally does not remit, and therefore definitive treatment is usually required. All patients are initially candidates for symptomatic treatment. β-blockers are usual therapy. Radioactive iodine therapy is recommended as first-line treatment for most non-pregnant, non-lactating patients. Doses are generally higher than those used for Graves' disease because toxic adenomas are more radioresistant.

332 J Surgery is the definitive management of thyroid cancer. Total thyroidectomy is indicated in patients who are older than 40 years with papillary carcinoma and in any patient with bilateral disease.

333 K Medullary cancer of the thyroid originates from the parafollicular cells (C cells) of the thyroid. It occurs in four clinical settings: sporadic, MEN type 2A, MEN 2B and inherited medullary carcinoma without associated endocrinopathies. All patients should receive total thyroidectomy, a complete central neck dissection and removal of all lymph nodes and surrounding fatty tissues within the side of the neck which harboured the tumour. Radioactive iodine therapy is not useful for the treatment of medullary thyroid cancer.

334 E Colloid nodules are the most common and do not have an increased risk of cancer.

335 C Radiotherapy is a standard treatment for lymphoma.

336 E Phenylketonuria is an autosomal recessive metabolic genetic disorder characterised by a deficiency in the hepatic enzyme phenylalanine hydroxylase. If the condition is left untreated, it can cause problems with brain development, leading to progressive mental retardation, brain damage and seizures.

337 B Gaucher's disease is the most common of the lysosomal storage diseases. It is caused by a hereditary deficiency of the enzyme glucocerebrosidase. Glucocerebroside can collect in the spleen, liver, kidneys, lungs, brain and bone marrow.

338 A McArdle's disease (myophosphorylase deficiency). The onset of this disease is usually noticed in childhood. A muscle biopsy will note the absence of myophosphorylase in muscle fibers.

339 F Galactosaemia follows an autosomal recessive mode of inheritance that confers a deficiency in an enzyme responsible for adequate galactose degradation. Galactosaemia is not related to and should not be confused with lactose intolerance. The only treatment for classic galactosaemia is eliminating lactose and galactose from the diet.

340 D Homocystinuria is an inherited disorder of the metabolism of the methionine, often involving cystathionine β-synthase. It is an inherited autosomal recessive trait.

341 J Cystinuria is an inherited autosomal recessive metabolic disorder that is characterised by the formation of cystine stones in the kidneys, ureter and bladder.

342 H Myasthenia gravis is an autoimmune neuromuscular disease leading to fluctuating muscle weakness and fatiguability. It is an autoimmune disorder in which weakness is caused by circulating antibodies that block acetylcholine receptors at the postsynaptic neuromuscular junction, inhibiting the stimulative effect of the acetylcholine. Myasthenia is treated medically with cholinesterase inhibitors or immunosuppressants, and, in selected cases, thymectomy.

343 F Diagnosis of Arnold–Chiari malformation is made through a combination of patient history, neurological examination and MRI.

344 A Multiple sclerosis is an inflammatory disease in which myelin sheaths in the brain and spinal cord are damaged, leading to demyelination and scarring, as well as a broad spectrum of signs and symptoms. During symptomatic attacks, administration of high doses of intravenous methylprednisolone is the routine therapy for acute relapses. Consequences of severe attacks which do not respond to corticosteroids might be treated by plasmapheresis. Disease modifying treatments include interferon, glatiramer, mitoxantrone and natalizumab.

345 G NPH is a chronic type of communicating hydrocephalus whereby the increase in intracranial pressure due to accumulation of cerebrospinal fluid becomes stable and the formation of CSF equilibrates with absorption. Because of this equilibration, patients do not exhibit the classic signs of increased intracranial pressure, such as nausea, vomiting, headache or impaired consciousness. Patients exhibit the classic triad of gait difficulties, urinary incontinence and mental decline.

346 I HSE is an acute or subacute illness, causing both general and focal signs of cerebral dysfunction. Although the presence of fever, headache, behavioural changes, confusion, focal neurological findings and abnormal CSF findings are suggestive of HSE, no pathognomonic clinical findings reliably distinguish HSE from other neurological disorders with similar presentations.

347 E Forms of motor neurone disease include amyotrophic lateral sclerosis, primary lateral sclerosis, progressive muscular atrophy, pseudobulbar palsy and progressive bulbar palsy. Symptoms usually present themselves between the ages of 50–70 years, and include progressive weakness, muscle wasting, and muscle fasciculations, spasticity or stiffness in the arms and legs and overactive tendon reflexes. Patients may present with symptoms as diverse as a dragging foot, unilateral muscle wasting in the hands or slurred speech.

348 D Interstitial nephritis is usually due to infection or reaction to medication. When caused by an allergic reaction, the symptoms of acute tubulointerstitial nephritis are fever, rash and enlarged kidneys. Some patients experience dysuria and lower back pain.

349 J Most patients with systemic lupus erythematosus (SLE) develop lupus nephritis early in their disease course. SLE is more common among women in the third decade of life, and lupus nephritis typically occurs in patients aged 20–40 years. Symptoms related to active nephritis may include peripheral oedema secondary to hypertension or hypoalbuminaemia. Laboratory abnormalities such as elevated serum creatinine levels, low albumin levels or urinary protein or sediment suggest active lupus nephritis.

350 A Medullary sponge kidney is a congenital disorder that can affect one or both kidneys, or only part of one kidney. There are ectatic and cystic changes of the medullary and papillary collecting ducts. Although it is a congenital disorder, diagnosis is often not made until the second or third decades, and it may be asymptomatic. Haematuria is common and usually microscopic, although macroscopic haematuria can occur with associated infection or calculi. Renal calculi may occur and are usually calcium oxalate and calcium phosphate. Recurrent urinary tract infection is a common presentation and affects more women than men. There may also be sterile pyuria.

351 F Hypercalciuria can be classified as idiopathic or secondary. Idiopathic hypercalciuria can be diagnosed when clinical, laboratory and radiographic investigations fail to delineate an underlying cause. Idiopathic hypercalciuria is the most common metabolic abnormality in patients with calcium kidney stones. Hypercalciuria can occur at any age, including newborns. The peak incidence of idiopathic hypercalciuria is in children aged 4–8 years.

352 H Cystinuria is an inherited autosomal recessive metabolic disorder that is characterised by the formation of cystine stones in the kidneys, ureter and bladder. Cystine stones are common in the second or third decade of life. The peak age of first renal calculus is 22 years.

353 B In RTA, an accumulation of acid in the body occurs due to a failure of the kidneys to appropriately acidify the urine. The metabolic acidosis that results from RTA may be caused either by failure to recover sufficient bicarbonate ions from the filtrate in the proximal tubule or by insufficient secretion of hydrogen ions into the distal tubule.

354 C Renal ultrasound is very good for showing hydronephrosis, renal stones, tumours or cysts. It provides important information regarding kidney function and is usually one of the first tests performed during an evaluation. Patients are advised to have a full bladder for the test.

355 B MRI has many advantages over CT in the examination of the brainstem and the posterior cranial fossa.

356 G Lumbar puncture in the presence of increased intracranial pressure may cause uncal herniation.

357 H Spiral (helical) CT scan has the advantage of being non-invasive, unlike the gold standard pulmonary angiogram.

358 D Duplex scanning with colour flow imaging provides instant visualisation of the veins and blood flow. It can detect the presence of both recent and old thrombi. In symptomatic patients the accuracy of duplex is 98% for iliac, femoral and popliteal thrombi and 90% for calf thrombi.

359 A Bone scans use radionuclides to detect areas of the bone which are growing or being repaired. Cells which are most 'active' in the target tissue or organ will take up more of the radionuclide. So, active parts of the tissue will emit more gamma rays than less active or inactive parts.

360 A A succenturiate (accessory) lobe is a second or third placental lobe that is much smaller than the largest lobe. Unlike bipartite lobes, the smaller succenturiate lobe often has areas of infarction or atrophy. The risk factors associated are advanced maternal age, primigravida, proteinuria in the first trimester of pregnancy, and major malformations in the foetus. The membranes between the lobes in such placenta can be torn during delivery, and the extra lobe can be retained after the rest of the placenta has been delivered, with consequent post-partum bleeding.

361 C A uterine rupture typically occurs during early labour, but may already develop during late pregnancy. A uterine scar from a previous Caesarean section is the most common risk factor. Other risk factors include myomectomy, dysfunctional labour, labour augmentation by oxytocin or prostaglandins, and high parity.

362 J Atonic uterus is failure of the uterus to contract with normal strength, duration and intervals during childbirth.

363 D The early stages of cervical cancer may be completely asymptomatic. Human papillomavirus (HPV) infection with high-risk types has been shown to be a necessary factor in the development of cervical cancer. Other risk factors include smoking, HIV infection, chlamydia infection, stress, dietary factors, hormonal contraception, multiple pregnancies and family history of cervical cancer. There is a possible genetic risk associated with *HLA*-B7.

364 C The initial signs and symptoms of uterine rupture are typically non-specific, which makes diagnosis difficult and sometimes delays definitive therapy. From the time of diagnosis to delivery, only 10–37 minutes are available before clinically significant foetal morbidity becomes inevitable. Foetal morbidity occurs as a result of catastrophic haemorrhage, foetal anoxia or both.

365 K Placenta accreta describes a condition where there is an abnormally deep attachment of the placenta, through the endometrium and into the myometrium. There are three forms of placenta accreta, distinguishable by the depth of penetration. The placenta usually detaches from the uterine wall relatively easily, but placenta accreta may cause haemorrhage during its removal. Accordingly, it commonly requires surgery.

366 H Placenta praevia involves implantation of the placenta over the internal cervical os. Variants include complete implantation over the os (complete placenta praevia), a placental edge partially covering the os (partial placenta praevia) or the placenta approaching the border of the os (marginal placenta praevia).

367 D Indications of D&C:
- evacuation of retained products of conception
- to treat intermenstrual bleeding
  ‣ to investigate the causes of infertility
  ‣ to remove polyps in the endometrial or inner lining of the uterus
  ‣ to diagnose endometrial cancer
  ‣ to remove an embedded intrauterine device used for contraception.
- to perform abortion in the early stages of pregnancy (though this is rare nowadays)
  ‣ to evacuate spontaneous abortion products
  ‣ to investigate the cause of abnormal bleeding in postmenopausal women taking HRT.

368 D D&C is usually a safe and simple procedure, and associated complications are rare, occurring in less than 5% of cases. However, possible complications could include uterine infection, haemorrhage and Asherman's syndrome.

369 B The most likely diagnosis here is polycystic ovaries. Accordingly, this young lady is a candidate for the combined oral contraceptive pill as it would regulate her periods and help reduce her blood loss. While she is anaemic, and would most probably benefit from iron supplements, it is more important at this stage to control her bleeding.

370 G Tranexamic acid can decrease dysfunctional uterine bleeding, probably through inhibition of prostaglandin synthesis. Once bleeding is controlled, tranexamic acid need only be used during menstruation.

371 C The presence of a fibroid does not mean that it needs to be removed. Excision is needed when the fibroid causes pain, pressure, abnormal bleeding or infertility.

372 A Indications for obtaining an endometrial biopsy in a non-pregnant woman include infertility, suspected uterine cancer, chronic anovulation (e.g. polycystic ovarian syndrome), and abnormal vaginal bleeding (e.g. endometrial hyperplasia or cancer).

373 A Aorto-femoral bypass is also called aorto-bifemoral bypass, since the new graft is formed in the shape of an upside-down 'y', with the top part attaching to the aorta and the lower parts attaching to each of the femoral arteries.

374 B Percutaneous transluminal angioplasty is a minimally invasive procedure used to open the blocked or narrowed femoral artery and to restore arterial blood flow to the lower leg. A catheter is inserted into the femoral artery. The catheter has a tiny balloon at its tip. The balloon is inflated once the catheter has been placed into the narrowed area of the artery. The inflation of the balloon compresses the fatty tissue in the artery and makes a larger opening inside the artery for improved blood flow. A stent may be inserted into the newly opened area of the artery to help keep the artery from narrowing or closing again.

375 H Femoro-tibial bypass is surgery to reroute blood from the femoral artery to the tibial artery in patients with severe peripheral artery disease. The saphenous vein in the leg or a synthetic graft is used for bypass.

376 D This is the insertion of a synthetic graft between the femoral arteries in both groins. Prognostic factors included poor run-off and distal disease, donor iliac artery stenosis prior to femoro-femoral bypass grafting, and progression of disease in the donor vessel following surgery.

377 D Multiple spinal sclerotic bone lesions are usually due to metastases. Other causes of sclerotic lesions include haemangioma, infarct, osteomyelitis, hyperparathyroidism and Paget's disease.

378 E Multiple myeloma is a cancer of plasma cells. Typical biochemical features include hypercalcaemia, anaemia, significantly raised ESR and urinary Bence Jones proteins.

379 A Osteosarcoma is an aggressive cancer arising from primitive transformed cells of mesenchymal origin that exhibit osteoblastic differentiation and produce malignant osteoid. It is the most common histological form of primary bone cancer. It usually develops during the period of rapid growth that occurs in adolescence, as a teenager matures into an adult. Complete radical surgical resection is the treatment of choice in osteosarcoma.

380 F Primary hyperparathyroidism results from over-secretion of PTH due to adenoma, hyperplasia or carcinoma of the parathyroid glands. PTH results in hypercalcaemia due to increased bone resorption, reduced renal clearance of calcium and increased intestinal calcium absorption.

381 A Rarely, Paget's disease is associated with the development of sarcoma. When there is a sudden onset or worsening of pain, sarcoma should be considered.

382 E Churg–Strauss syndrome is a medium and small vessel autoimmune vasculitis leading to necrosis. It involves mainly the blood vessels of the lungs (where it may begin as a severe asthma), gastrointestinal system, peripheral nerves, heart, skin and kidneys. Diagnostic markers include eosinophil granulocytes and granulomas in affected tissue and anti-neutrophil cytoplasmic antibodies (ANCA) against neutrophil granulocytes. Differentiation from Wegener's granulomatosis is simple, as Wegener's is closely associated with c-ANCA, while Churg–Strauss shows elevations of p-ANCA.

383 I Goodpasture's syndrome (anti-glomerular basement antibody disease) is a rare condition characterised by glomerulonephritis and pulmonary haemorrhage. Because of the vagueness of early symptoms and rapid progression of the disease, diagnosis is often not reached until very late in the course of the disease. A kidney biopsy (linear IgG deposits along basement membrane) is often the fastest way to explore the diagnosis, the extent of the disease and likely effect of treatment. Tests for anti-GBM antibodies may also be useful, combined with tests for antibodies to neutrophil cytoplasmic antigens.

384 G ABPA is characterised by a hypersensitivity response to *Aspergillus* (most commonly *A. fumigatus*). It occurs most often in patients with asthma or cystic fibrosis. Diagnosis is usually achieved using chest X-rays, CT scans, raised blood levels of IgE and eosinophils, immunological tests for *Aspergillus* together with sputum staining and sputum cultures. Treatment consists of corticosteroids and antifungal medications.

385 A EAA is an inflammation of the alveoli caused by hypersensitivity to inhaled organic dusts. It is categorised as acute, subacute and chronic, based on the duration of the illness. The diagnosis is based upon a history of symptoms after exposure to the allergen, chest X-ray and spirometry, which typically shows a restrictive pattern.

386 C Accentuated second heart sound reflects pulmonary hypertension, which is a complication of CFA.

387 K Pulmonary embolism is a serious complication of any operation in view of the resulting poor mobility, which may precipitate DVT resulting in pulmonary embolism.

388 C Bartter's syndrome is a rare inherited defect in the thick ascending limb of the loop of Henle. It is characterised by hypokalaemia, alkalosis, elevated renin and aldosterone levels, and normal to low blood pressure, i.e. identical symptoms to those of patients who are on loop diuretics, e.g. furosemide.

389 J Rhabdomyolysis is the rapid destruction of skeletal muscle resulting in myoglobinuria. It can be caused by severe muscle contractions from prolonged seizures.

390 F Nephrotic syndrome is a non-specific renal pathology resulting in proteinuria of at least 3.5 g per day per 1.73 m^2 body surface area, resulting in hypoalbuminaemia, hyperlipidaemia and oedema. In nephrotic syndrome, there are small pores in the podocytes, large enough to permit proteinuria but not large enough to allow cells through, hence no haematuria. By contrast, in nephritic syndrome, RBCs pass through the pores, causing haematuria.

391 G Alport syndrome (hereditary nephritis) is a genetic disorder characterised by glomerulonephritis, end-stage kidney disease and hearing loss. Alport syndrome can also affect the eyes, resulting in lenticonus. Haematuria is characteristic.

392 A Although renal vein thrombosis has numerous causes, it occurs most commonly in patients with nephrotic syndrome, as in this patient, who has evidence of fluid overload and right pleural effusion. Renal ultrasound is a safe non-invasive technique. With underlying renal vein thrombosis, the kidneys swell and become echogenic, with prominent echo-poor medullary pyramids. However, ultrasound is usually not sensitive enough to assist in making the diagnosis. CT scan is the current procedure of choice for diagnosing renal vein thrombosis non-invasively.

393 E RTA is a condition that involves an accumulation of acid in the body due to failure of the kidneys to appropriately acidify the urine. Several types of RTA exist, which all have different syndromes and different causes. The metabolic acidosis caused by RTA is a normal anion gap acidosis.

394 B The post-coital test is generally done a day or two prior to ovulation. It is considered normal if there are normal amounts of sperm in the sample, sperm is moving forward through the cervical mucous, the mucous stretches at least 2 in (spinnbarkeit) and the mucous dries in a fern-like pattern.

395 D A normal HSG result shows the filling of the uterine cavity and the bilateral filling of the fallopian tube with the contrast.

396 I Laparoscopy is the most common surgical procedure for the diagnosis and treatment of endometriosis.

397 K Chlamydia infection is the most common sexually transmitted disease in the UK. Nucleic acid amplification tests (NAAT), such as polymerase chain reaction (PCR), transcription-mediated amplification (TMA) and DNA strand displacement amplification (SDA), are now the mainstays. NAAT for chlamydia may be performed on swab specimens collected from the cervix (women) or urethra (men), on self-collected vaginal swabs or on voided urine. Urine and self-collected swab testing facilitates the performance of screening tests in settings where genital examination is impractical.

398 H Changes in both the amount and texture of cervical mucus are indicators of ovulation (fertile window).

399 H If a pregnant woman is identified as being infected with syphilis, treatment can effectively prevent congenital syphilis from developing in the unborn child, especially if she is treated before the 16th week of pregnancy. The child is at greatest risk of contracting syphilis when the mother is in the early stages of infection, but the disease can be passed at any point during pregnancy, even during delivery (should the child not have contracted it already).

400 C Most congenitally infected children do not have symptoms. Only 10% of infants congenitally infected with CMV are symptomatic. There is no specific treatment for congenital CMV.

401 A Cardiovascular anomalies are associated with Coxsackie B3 and B4 infection during pregnancy. The likelihood of congenital heart disease is increased by maternal infection with two or more Coxsackie B viruses rather than one.

402 J Congenital rubella syndrome can occur in a developing foetus of a pregnant woman who has contracted rubella during her first trimester. If infection occurs 0–28 days before conception, there is a 43% chance the infant will be affected. If the infection occurs 0–12 weeks after conception, there is a 51% chance the infant will be affected. If the infection occurs 13–26 weeks after conception, there is a 23% chance the infant will be affected by the disease. Infants are not generally affected if rubella is contracted during the third trimester, or 26–40 weeks after conception. Problems rarely occur when rubella is contracted by the mother after 20 weeks of gestation and continues to disseminate the virus after birth.

403 E Up to half of the foetuses who become infected with toxoplasmosis during pregnancy are born prematurely. Often, there are signs of infection in the baby at birth. However, newborns with milder infections may not have symptoms or problems for months or even years.

404 F Foetal exposure to mumps rarely proves to be a problem, although there have been cases of spontaneous abortion and endocardial fibroelastosis. Infection late in the pregnancy can result in the infant contracting mumps.

405 B De Quervain's (subacute granulomatous) thyroiditis is the most common cause of a painful thyroid gland. It is a transient inflammation of the thyroid, the clinical course of which is highly variable. Most patients have pain in the region of the thyroid, which is usually diffusely tender, and some have systemic symptoms. Hyperthyroidism often occurs initially, sometimes followed by transient hypothyroidism. Complete recovery in weeks to months is characteristic.

406 D MEN type 1 is an inherited disorder in which one or more of the endocrine glands are overactive or form a tumour. Endocrine glands most commonly involved include the pancreas, parathyroid and pituitary.

407 C Those are typical symptoms of hypothyroidism.

408 G Graves' disease is an autoimmune disease caused by autoantibodies to the TSH receptor which activate that TSH receptor, thereby stimulating thyroid hormone synthesis and secretion, and a diffusely enlarged goitre.

409 A A thyroglossal cyst is a fibrous cyst that forms from a persistent thyroglossal duct. It usually presents as a midline neck lump which is painless, smooth and cystic. It moves upwards with protrusion of the tongue.

410 F Hashimoto's thyroiditis (chronic lymphocytic thyroiditis) is an autoimmune disease in which the thyroid gland is gradually destroyed by a variety of cell and antibody-mediated immune processes. It is usually treated with levothyroxine. It is recommended that the TSH levels be kept under 3.

411 H Toxoplasmosis is a parasitic disease caused by *Toxoplasma gondii*. Although cats are often blamed for spreading toxoplasmosis, contact with raw meat is a more significant source of human infections in many countries, and faecal contamination of hands is a greater risk factor. During the first few weeks post exposure, the infection typically causes a mild flu-like illness or no illness. Thereafter, the parasite rarely causes any symptoms in otherwise healthy adults. However, those with a weakened immune system, such as AIDS patients or pregnant women, may become seriously ill, and it can occasionally be fatal. The parasite can cause encephalitis and neurologic diseases (e.g. brain abscess), and can affect the heart, liver, inner ears and eyes (chorioretinitis).

412 B Lyme disease is a tick-borne disease. Early symptoms may include fever, headache, fatigue, depression and a characteristic circular skin rash (erythema migrans). If it is untreated, later symptoms may involve the joints, heart and central nervous system. In most cases, the infection and its symptoms are eliminated by antibiotics, especially if the illness is treated early. Antibiotics of choice are doxycycline (in adults), amoxicillin (in children), erythromycin (for pregnant women) and ceftriaxone, with treatment lasting 10–28 days.

413 E Trichinosis is a parasitic disease caused by eating raw or undercooked pork or wild game infected with the larvae of *Trichinella spiralis*. The case definition for trichinosis at the European Centre for Disease Prevention and Control states 'at least three of the following six: fever, muscle soreness and pain, gastrointestinal symptoms, facial oedema, eosinophilia, subconjunctival, subungual, and retinal haemorrhages'.

414 J Leishmaniasis is a disease caused by *Leishmania* and is transmitted by the bite of the sandfly. Most forms of the disease are transmissible only from animals, but some can be spread between humans. Cutaneous leishmaniasis is the most common form of leishmaniasis. Visceral leishmaniasis (kala-azar) is a severe form in which the parasites have migrated to the vital organs. The most typical symptoms are fever, splenomegaly and hepatomegaly. It is diagnosed in the haematology laboratory by direct visualisation of the Leishman–Donovan bodies.

415 G Leptospirosis (Weil's disease), is caused by spirochaetes of the genus *Leptospira*. It is usually transmitted to humans by allowing water that has been contaminated by animal urine to come in contact with unhealed breaks in the skin, the eyes or with the mucous membranes. Outside of tropical areas, leptospirosis cases have a relatively distinct seasonality, with most of them occurring at early spring and early autumn. It is a biphasic disease that begins with flu-like symptoms. The first phase resolves, and the patient is briefly asymptomatic until the second phase begins, which is characterised by meningitis, jaundice and renal failure.

416 C Toxic shock syndrome is caused by toxins of *Staphylococcus aureus* or *Streptococcus pyogenes*. There is a connection between toxic shock syndrome and tampon use.

417 B Such a history of alcoholism, rapid weight loss and dysphagia points towards a malignancy. The most likely cause is oesophageal cancer, in view of the progressive dysphagia, which is typically to solids.

418 I A pharyngeal pouch is a pulsion diverticulum of the pharyngeal mucosa through Killian's dehiscence, an area of weakness between the two parts of the inferior pharyngeal constrictor – the thyropharyngeus and the cricopharyngeus – at their posterior margin. The pouch probably arises as a result of a relative obstruction at the level of the cricopharyngeus. At first, it develops posteriorly, but then it protrudes to one side, usually the left. As it enlarges, it displaces the oesophagus laterally.

419 A About eight in 10 salivary stones form in one of the submandibular glands. Diagnosis is usually made by characteristic history and physical examination. Diagnosis can be confirmed by X-ray (80% of salivary gland calculi are visible on X-ray), or by sialogram or ultrasound.

420 D Achalasia is an oesophageal motility disorder involving the smooth muscle layer of the oesophagus and the lower oesophageal sphincter. It is characterised by difficulty swallowing, regurgitation and sometimes chest pain. Diagnosis is reached with oesophageal manometry and barium swallow studies.

421 L This is a classic presentation of acute diverticulitis. It is worth noting that most people with diverticulosis are asymptomatic, though symptoms may include mild cramps, bloating and constipation.

422 D Surgery is the mainstay of treatment for thymoma. If the tumour is apparently invasive and large, preoperative chemotherapy may be used to decrease the size and improve resectability before surgery is attempted.

423 E All thymomas should be considered as malignant, as even the encapsulated ones may recur and metastasise.

424 G Acetylcholinesterase inhibitors, e.g. neostigmine and pyridostigmine, can improve muscle function by slowing the natural enzyme cholinesterase that degrades acetylcholine in the motor end plate; the neurotransmitter is therefore around longer to stimulate its receptor.

425 E Thymoma is relatively rare in younger (< 40 years old) patients, but paradoxically younger patients with generalised myasthenia gravis without thymoma benefit from thymectomy. Resection is also indicated for those with a thymoma, but it is less likely to improve the myasthenia gravis symptoms.

426 K If the myasthenia is serious (myasthenic crisis), plasmapheresis can be used to remove the putative antibody from the circulation. Also, intravenous immunoglobulins (IVIG) can be used to bind the circulating antibodies. Both of these treatments have relatively short-lived benefits, typically measured in weeks.

427 E The limited cutaneous form of systemic sclerosis scleroderma is often referred to as CREST syndrome. CREST is an acronym for the five main features: **C**alcinosis, **R**aynaud's syndrome, o**E**sophageal dysmotility, **S**clerodactyly and **T**elangiectasia.

428 I Reiter's syndrome is characterised by a triad of arthritis, non-gonococcal urethritis and conjunctivitis, and by lesions of the skin and mucosal surfaces.

429 B GCA (temporal arteritis) is a form of vasculitis most commonly involving large and medium arteries of the head. The disorder may coexist with polymyalgia rheumatica.

430 F Some physicians make a diagnosis on the basis of the American College of Rheumatology classification criteria. The criteria, however, were established mainly for use in scientific research, including use in randomised controlled trials which require higher confidence levels, so some people with SLE may not pass the full criteria. However, in clinical practice SLE is diagnosed if a person has an immunologic disorder (anti-DNA antibody, anti-Smith antibody, false positive syphilis test, or LE cells) or malar rash. It has sensitivity = 92% and specificity = 92%.

431 D Polymyositis is a type of chronic inflammatory myopathy related to dermatomyositis. It tends to become evident in adulthood, presenting with bilateral proximal muscle weakness often noted in the upper legs due to early fatigue while walking. Diagnosis is fourfold, including elevation of creatine kinase, history and physical examination, EMG changes, and a positive muscle biopsy. Anti-Jo antibodies are present in > 65% of patients.

432 K Sjögren's syndrome (Sicca syndrome) is a systemic autoimmune disease affecting the exocrine glands. Ninety per cent of Sjögren's patients are women and the average age of onset is late 40s. It can exist as a disorder in its own right (primary Sjögren's syndrome) or it may develop years after the onset of an associated rheumatic disorder (secondary Sjögren's syndrome). Typical Sjögren's syndrome ANA patterns are SSA/Ro and SSB/La, of which SSB/La is far more specific. SSA/Ro is associated with numerous other autoimmune conditions but is often present in Sjögren's. Schirmer's test can be used to measure the production of tears.

433 B Gonorrhoea usually presents in men with dysuria and penile discharge. Women, on the other hand, are asymptomatic (50% of cases) or have vaginal discharge and pelvic pain.

434 D Lymphogranuloma venereum is a sexually transmitted disease caused by *Chlamydia trachomatis*. It is primarily an infection of lymphatics and lymph nodes. Chlamydia gains entrance through breaks in the skin, or it can cross the epithelial cell layer of mucous membranes. Spontaneous remission is common. Complete cure can be obtained with proper antibiotics, such as tetracycline, doxycycline or erythromycin.

435 G Although genital herpes is largely believed to be caused by HSV-2, genital HSV-1 infections are increasing and now exceed 50% in certain populations.

436 H *Gardnerella* is a Gram-variable-staining, anaerobic bacteria that can cause bacterial vaginosis in some women as a result of a disruption in the normal vaginal microflora. It can be treated with metronidazole.

437 I *Chlamydia trachomatis* is an obligate intracellular pathogen. Both sexes can display urethritis, proctitis, trachoma and infertility. In men, it can cause prostatitis and epididymitis. In women, it can cause cervicitis, pelvic inflammatory disease, ectopic pregnancy and acute or chronic pelvic pain.

438 J Trichomoniasis is a sexually transmitted infection of the urogenital tract. The most common site of infection is the urethra and the vagina in women. The infection is more likely to occur if the normal pH of the vagina is shifted from a healthy semi-acidic (3.8–4.2) to a much more alkaline one (5–6) that is conducive to *T. vaginalis* growth. Men with this infection rarely exhibit symptoms.

439 A Danazol was approved by the US Food and Drug Administration as the first drug to specifically treat endometriosis in the early 1970s. Its use is now limited by its masculinising side effects.

440 D A GnRH agonist activates the GnRH receptor resulting in increased secretion of FSH and LH. GnRH agonists are used in treatment of cancers that are hormonally sensitive, e.g. prostate cancer and breast cancer, IVF therapy, some cases of congenital adrenal hyperplasia, and in women with menorrhagia, endometriosis, adenomyosis or uterine fibroids (to suppress ovarian activity and induce a hypo-oestrogenic state).

441 G Relatively common side effects of progestogens include acne, dizziness, drowsiness, headache, hot flashes and nausea, in addition to irregular periods.

442 B Clomiphene is used to induce ovulation in cases of infertility.

443 H Taking HRT can make a huge difference to a woman's quality of life and well-being. HRT can also reduce a woman's risk of developing osteoporosis and cancer of the colon and rectum. However, the long-term use of HRT to prevent osteoporosis is not usually recommended. This is because HRT slightly increases the risk of developing breast cancer, endometrial cancer, ovarian cancer and stroke. In addition, there are other medications available for osteoporosis that do not carry the same level of associated risk.

444 F Bromocriptine is a dopamine agonist that is used in the treatment of pituitary tumours, hyperprolactinaemia, Parkinson's disease and neuroleptic malignant syndrome.

445 B Lactational mastitis/breast abscess occurs 2–3 weeks after nursing and is usually due to a cracked nipple. The most common organism is *Staphylococcus aureus*. It usually responds to a course of antibiotics. Patients are often advised to continue breastfeeding in order to promote drainage of the breast unless they drain frank pus or if they are HIV positive (as viral load may increase the mother-to-child transmission rate).

446 I Duct ectasia can mimic breast cancer, though it is an inflammatory condition involving the large subareolar ducts. It is a disorder of premenopausal age. Features of duct ectasia can include nipple retraction, inversion, pain and sometimes bloody discharge. It can be difficult to distinguish from intraductal papilloma, but in ductal ectasia, cytology of the discharge shows macrophages and debris rather than epithelial cells in the case of intraductal papilloma.

447 C Fibroadenosis (fibrocystic disease) is the most common cause of breast lumps in women of reproductive age. The peak incidence is between 35–50 years of age. It is rare before the age of 25. It is related to an imbalance between oestrogens and progesterone during each menstrual cycle. It is characterised by overgrowth of both fibrous stroma, and of epithelial elements, i.e. ducts and lobules, in differing proportions. Only in those cases showing marked epithelial hyperplasia (epitheliosis) is the risk of breast carcinoma thought to be increased.

448 E The main differential diagnosis for a mass with microcalcification is an invasive intraductal carcinoma and a radial scar. The presence of lymphadenopathy suggests an underlying malignancy. Ductal carcinomas constitute about 75% of cases of breast cancer while lobular carcinomas constitute about 10%.

449 A A fibroadenoma is a small, solid, rubbery, noncancerous, harmless lump composed of fibrous and glandular tissue. It is the most common benign breast tumour, occuring mainly in young women. The tumour contains glandular epithelium and connective tissue stroma. They are not attached to surrounding breast tissue, thus their mobility.

450 H Whipple's disease is a rare, systemic infectious disease caused by *Tropheryma whipplei*. The most common symptoms are diarrhoea, abdominal pain, weight loss and arthralgia. Occasionally, the joint pains occur many years before any digestive tract symptoms develop.

451 G Osteomalacia may be the only presenting feature of coeliac disease, so it should be considered in the differential diagnosis of patients presenting with proximal muscle weakness and diffuse musculoskeletal pain.

452 F Pancreatic cancer is sometimes called a 'silent killer' because early pancreatic cancer often does not cause symptoms, and the later symptoms are usually non-specific and varied. Severe abdominal pain radiating to the back should raise suspicion to the diagnosis of pancreatic cancer.

453 B Abdominal pain may be the initial symptom of Crohn's disease. It is often accompanied by diarrhoea, especially in those who have had surgery. The diarrhoea may or may not be bloody. In severe cases, an individual may have more than 20 bowel movements per day and may need to awaken at night to defecate. Crohn's disease can lead to several mechanical complications within the intestines, including obstruction, fistulae, abscesses, and increased risk of cancer in the area of inflammation.

454 C The clue in this question is the history of recurrent chest infections as well as the young age of the patient, which point towards cystic fibrosis.

455 A Patients with chronic pancreatitis usually present with persistent nausea, abdominal pain and/or steatorrhea. Diabetes is a common complication due to the chronic pancreatic damage and may require treatment with insulin. In developed countries, the most common cause is alcoholism.

456 H Coarctation of the aorta is a congenital condition whereby the aorta narrows in the area where the ligamentum arteriosum inserts. In mild cases, children may show no signs or symptoms at first, and their condition may not be diagnosed until later in life.

457 A Once a diagnosis of ASD is made, a decision has to be taken on whether it should be corrected. Surgical mortality due to closure of an ASD is lowest when the procedure is performed prior to the development of significant pulmonary hypertension. The lowest mortality rates are achieved in individuals with a pulmonary artery systolic pressure of less than 40 mmHg.

458 D VSD is usually asymptomatic at birth. It usually manifests a few weeks after birth. VSD is an acyanotic congenital heart defect (left-to-right shunt), so there are no signs of cyanosis. Most cases don't need treatment and heal at the first years of life. Treatment is either conservative or surgical. Smaller congenital VSDs often close on their own as the heart grows, and in such cases may be treated conservatively. Some cases may necessitate surgical intervention.

459 E A patent ductus arteriosus can be idiopathic or secondary to preterm birth, congenital rubella syndrome and chromosomal abnormalities, e.g. Down's syndrome. PDA may lead to congestive heart failure if left uncorrected.

460 G Fallot's tetralogy is the most common congenital cyanotic heart disease. It has the following features: right ventricular hypertrophy, VSD, pulmonary stenosis and overriding aorta.

461 B Ebstein's anomaly is a congenital malformation of the heart that is characterised by apical displacement of the septal and posterior tricuspid valve leaflets, leading to atrialisation of the right ventricle with a variable degree of malformation and displacement of the anterior leaflet.

462 G The most common cause of haematemesis is bleeding from a peptic ulcer. OGD identifies the cause in > 90% of cases and permits treatment, e.g. sclerotherapy for varices or injection of adrenaline into a bleeding ulcer.

463 D Mesenteric ischaemia can be difficult to diagnose in clinical practice. However, ischaemic events can be classified by the rapidity of symptom onset, the degree of impairment of blood flow, and the region of the bowel affected. Mesenteric angiography is the test of choice for the diagnosis of arterial causes of acute mesenteric ischaemia despite being expensive and invasive, in view of its usefulness as a diagnostic and therapeutic tool for lower gastrointestinal haemorrhage.

464 J This is a case of intestinal obstruction. Erect abdominal X-rays are requested to look for fluid levels in obstruction or ileus. Air under the diaphragm may be seen in an erect picture if the bowel has been perforated, although a chest X-ray is more usual to look for that sign.

465 I Those are classic features of cholecystitis. An ultrasound scan is the best investigation to confirm the diagnosis.

466 A Those features are suggestive of cancer at the head of the pancreas, which would be best investigated in this case with a CT scan.

467 F The middle cerebral artery arises from the internal carotid artery. Broca's area of speech lies at the lateroinferior frontal lobe.

468 K The posterior inferior cerebellar artery is the largest branch of the vertebral artery. A thrombus affecting this artery leads to lateral medullary syndrome (Wallenberg syndrome).

469 D The posterior cerebral artery arises from the basilar artery and supplies the occipital lobe.

470 B The anterior cerebral artery arises from the internal carotid artery and forms a part of the circle of Willis. Anterior cerebral artery occlusion results in paralysis or weakness of the contralateral foot and leg.

471 A The basilar artery arises from the confluence of the two vertebral arteries at the junction between the medulla oblongata and the pons. Basilar artery thrombosis is the most common cause of locked-in syndrome.

472 F The middle cerebral artery is by far the largest cerebral artery and is the vessel most commonly affected by cerebrovascular accident (CVA). It supplies most of the outer brain surface, nearly all the basal ganglia, and the posterior and anterior internal capsules.

473 B Pregnancy is a predisposing factor for pulmonary embolism. The family history of IHD in this case is irrelevant, as the symptoms (particularly cyanosis) are not compatible with a myocardial infarction.

474 J Musculoskeletal pain caused by cough is relatively common in clinical practice. Chest wall tenderness and lack of other physical signs point to the diagnosis.

475 A The history and examination hint at Marfan's syndrome, which may be associated with an aortic anuerysm.

476 I Substernal or left precordial pleuritic pain with radiation to the trapezius ridge, which is relieved by sitting up and bending forward and worsened by lying down or inspiration, is characteristic of pericarditis.

477 B Cigar cells are commonly associated with hereditary elliptocytosis, however they may also be seen in iron deficiency anaemia.

478 E Megaloblastic anaemia is most commonly due to deficiency of vitamin B_{12} and/or folic acid. Vitamin B_{12} deficiency alone will not cause megaloblastic anaemia in the presence of sufficient folate, for the mechanism is loss of B_{12}-dependent folate recycling, followed by folate-deficiency loss of nucleic acid synthesis (specifically thymine), leading to defects in DNA synthesis. Folic acid supplementation in the absence of vitamin B_{12} prevents this type of anaemia (although other vitamin B_{12}-specific pathologies continue).

479 J Target cells are associated with haemoglobin C disease, asplenia, liver disease, thalassaemia and severe iron deficiency anaemia.

480 F Sickle cell disease is an autosomal codominant blood disorder characterised by red blood cells that assume an abnormal, rigid, sickle shape.

481 I Myelofibrosis is a myeloproliferative disease in which the proliferation of an abnormal type of bone marrow stem cell results in fibrosis, or the replacement of the marrow with collagenous connective tissue fibers. The only known cure is allogeneic stem cell transplantation.

482 G Rouleaux formation is seen in infections, multiple myeloma, inflammatory and connective tissue disorders, cancers and diabetes mellitus. Abnormal plasma cells are seen in multiple myeloma.

483 J In osteoarthritis, Heberden's nodes (on the distal interphalangeal joints) and/or Bouchard's nodes (on the proximal interphalangeal joints) may form, though they are not necessarily painful.

484 I According to the American College of Rheumatology classification criteria for vasculitides, including polyarteritis nodosa (PAN), three of the following 10 criteria must be present to classify a vasculitis as PAN:
- weight loss of 4 kg or more
- livedo reticularis
- testicular pain/tenderness
- myalgia or leg weakness/tenderness
- mononeuropathy or polyneuropathy
- diastolic blood pressure greater than 90 mmHg
- elevated BUN and creatinine levels
- infection with hepatitis B virus
- abnormality on arteriography
- biopsy of small- or medium-sized artery containing polymorphonuclear neutrophils.

485 K Pseudogout is caused by deposits of calcium pyrophosphate crystals in and around the joints. It has been reported to occasionally coexist with gout. Pseudogout can result in arthritis of a number of joints but commonly involves the knees, wrists, shoulders, hips and/or ankles. It usually affects only one or a few joints at a time. Attacks of joint inflammation, characterised by acute joint swelling, warmth, stiffness and pain, may last for days to weeks and can resolve spontaneously. It is characterised by the presence of abnormal calcifications in cartilage of joints on X-rays (chondrocalcinosis).

486 A Most people with SLE will develop arthritis during the course of their illness. Arthritis in SLE commonly involves swelling, pain, stiffness and even deformity of the small joints of the hands, wrists and feet. Sometimes, the arthritis of SLE can mimic that of rheumatoid arthritis.

487 C Reiter's syndrome (reactive arthritis) most commonly strikes individuals aged 20–40 years, is more common in men than in women, and more common in whites than in blacks. This is owing to the high frequency of the *HLA*-B27 gene in the white population.

488 E Felty's syndrome is characterised by the combination of rheumatoid arthritis, splenomegaly and neutropenia.

489 B In Addison's disease, hyperkalaemia and hyponatraemia are due to aldosterone deficiency while hypoglycaemia is due to loss of glucocorticoid's glucogenic effect.

490 H Pyloric stenosis results in vomiting, causing loss of hydrogen ions.

491 E Cushing's disease results in metabolic changes opposite to those of Addison's disease.

492 J In multiple myeloma, hypercalcaemia is due to osteoclastic activity.

493 D Small cell (oat cell) carcinoma may be associated with SIADH, which results in hyponatraemia.

494 A Those are typical features of primary hypoparathyroidism.

495 C L4 also supplies the knee caps.

496 A C8 supplies the fourth and fifth fingers, C7 supplies the second and third fingers dorsally and ventrally, and C6 supplies the thumb and index finger.

497 I S1 has a large distribution over the gluteal region, back of the thigh and leg, extending into the lateral aspect of the foot.

498 G T10 characteristically supplies the umbilicus (relevant to appendicitis, as the pain may begin around the umbilicus).

499 E T1 also supplies a segment across the chest and the back. T4 supplies the nipples.

500 J L5 also supplies the lateral aspect of the thigh and the anterior aspect of the leg.

501 K The accessory nerve (XI) controls sternocleidomastoid and trapezius muscles and overlaps with functions of the vagus.

502 L The hypoglossal nerve (XII) provides motor innervation to the muscles of the tongue (except for the palatoglossus, which is innervated by the vagus) and other glossal muscles.

503 I The glossopharyngeal nerve (IX) receives taste from the posterior third of the tongue, provides secretomotor innervation to the parotid gland, and provides motor innervation to the stylopharyngeus.

504 E The trigeminal nerve (V) receives sensation from the face and innervates the muscles of mastication.

505 D The trochlear nerve (IV) innervates the superior oblique muscle, which depresses, rotates laterally and intorts the eyeball.

506 F The abducens nerve (VI) innervates the lateral rectus, which abducts the eye.

507 F Diagnosis of meningococcal meningitis is by detection of cryptococcal antigen by culture of CSF. Blood cultures may be positive in heavy infections.

508 B Kaposi's sarcoma commonly affects the lower limbs, back, face, mouth and genitalia.

509 E Progressive multifocal leucoencephalopathy is characterised by progressive damage or inflammation of the white matter of the brain at multiple locations.

510 I A growing space-occupying lesion in the brain, e.g. lymphoma, typically presents with progressive neurological deficit, e.g. progressive hemiparesis.

511 A Numbness, tingling and pain are well-recognised features of polyneuropathy.

512 C MRI is considered superior to CT scanning in the detection of brain toxoplasmosis. The administration of IV contrast material with either modality improves the diagnostic yield and accuracy.

513 F TR is most commonly caused by dilation of the right ventricle with malfunction of a normal valve, as occurs in pulmonary hypertension, RV dysfunction-induced heart failure and pulmonary outflow tract obstruction.

514 A About half of the cases of aortic insufficiency are due to aortic root dilatation, which is idiopathic in over 80% of cases, but otherwise may result from ageing, syphilitic aortitis, osteogenesis imperfecta, aortic dissection, Behçet's disease, reactive arthritis and systemic hypertension. In about 15% the cause is innate bicuspid aortic valve, while another 15% of cases are due to retraction of the cusps as part of post-inflammatory processes of endocarditis in rheumatic fever and various collagen vascular diseases. Hill's sign refers to a ≥ 20 mmHg difference in popliteal and brachial systolic cuff pressures, and is seen in chronic severe aortic regurgitation.

515 G Mitral valve prolapse is characterised by the displacement of an abnormally thickened mitral valve leaflet into the left atrium during systole. Most cases carry a low risk of complications. Complications include mitral regurgitation, infective endocarditis, congestive heart failure and, rarely, sudden death due to cardiac arrest.

516 D Second heart sound is normally split in mild aortic stenosis, P_2 preceding A_2. As stenosis increases in severity, then reversed splitting occurs, i.e. A_2 preceding P_2. If there is calcification of the aortic valve, then A_2 will become softer and may be inaudible all together.

517 I In mitral stenosis, the first heart sound is unusually loud and may be palpable (tapping apex beat) because of increased force in closing the mitral valve.

518 B In HCM, if dynamic outflow obstruction exists, physical examination findings may include pulsus bisferiens and double apical impulse with each ventricular contraction. These findings, when present, can help differentiate HCM from aortic stenosis.

519 C Warfarin-induced skin necrosis (WISN) is a potentially catastrophic complication of warfarin therapy in patients with protein C deficiency that arises as a result of the different half-lives of the vitamin K-dependent proteins. One day after initiation of warfarin, protein C activity is reduced by approximately 50%. Owing to their longer half-lives, the levels of the vitamin K-dependent clotting factors II, IX and X decline more slowly. The reduced level of protein C activity relative to these other procoagulant molecules creates a transient hypercoagulable state. WISN typically occurs during the first few days of warfarin therapy, often when daily doses in excess of 10 mg are administered.

520 H Trousseau syndrome is associated with certain cancers, where there is venous thrombosis and hypercoagulability. It is typically associated with adenocarcinoma of the pancreas or the lungs. In this case, there are several clues regarding lung cancer (old, male, smoker, with prolonged cough and haemoptysis).

521 E Antiphospholipid antibody syndrome is a coagulation disorder resulting in thrombosis in arteries and veins as well as pregnancy-related complications (due to thrombi within the placenta), e.g. miscarriage, stillbirth, preterm delivery or severe pre-eclampsia. It is due to the production of antibodies against phospholipids in cell membrane. In particular, the disease is characterised by antibodies against cardiolipin and β_2-glycoprotein I.

522 A PNH is a rare, acquired, potentially life-threatening disease characterised by complement-induced intravascular haemolytic anaemia, haemoglobinuria and thrombosis. Ham's acid haemolysis test is the classic test for PNH, but more modern tests include flow cytometry for CD55 and CD59 on white and red blood cells.

523 B Thrombotic thrombocytopenic purpura results in extensive microscopic thromboses in small blood vessels throughout the body (thrombotic microangiopathy). Plasmapheresis is currently the treatment of choice for TTP. However, most patients with refractory or relapsing TTP receive additional immunosuppressive therapy.

524 I Waldenström's macroglobulinaemia is characterised by an uncontrolled clonal proliferation of terminally differentiated B lymphocytes. Symptoms include flu-like symptoms, weight loss and chronic nasal and gingival bleeding. Peripheral neuropathy can occur in 10% of patients. Lymphadenopathy, splenomegaly, and/or hepatomegaly are present in 30%–40% of cases. Some symptoms are due to the effects of the IgM paraprotein, which may cause cryoglobulinaemia. Other symptoms are due to the hyperviscosity syndrome, which is present in 6%–20% of patients. This is attributed to the IgM monoclonal protein increasing the viscosity of the blood. Symptoms of this are mainly neurologic and can include blurring or loss of vision, headache and, rarely, stroke or coma.

525 I Collagenous colitis has a peak incidence in the fifth decade of life, affecting women more than men. It typically presents with watery diarrhoea, usually in the absence of rectal bleeding. Biopsies of affected tissue usually show deposition of collagen in the lamina propria.

526 F *Campylobacter* is the most common reported bacterial cause of infectious intestinal disease in the UK. The incubation period can be 1–11 days but is usually 2–5 days. There is a prodromal illness of fever, headache and myalgia lasting up to 24 hours. The fever may be as high as 40°C and fever, whether high or low, may persist for a week. There are abdominal pains and cramps, and profuse diarrhoea with up to 10 stools a day. The stool is watery and often bloody.

527 D Laxative abuse is rather common in clinical practice. In young females, it is frequently associated with attempts to lose weight. In this case, hospital admission (where the patient has no access to laxatives) seemed to favour the diagnosis.

528 B The main symptom of active ulcerative colitis is usually constant diarrhoea mixed with blood, of gradual onset. Its peak incidence is between 15–25 years. Ulcerative colitis is normally continuous from the rectum up the colon.

529 G Pseudomembranous colitis is a cause of antibiotic-associated diarrhoea. It is often caused by *Clostridium difficile*. It is characterised by offensive-smelling diarrhoea, fever and abdominal pain.

530 J IBS is a diagnosis of exclusion. It is a functional bowel disorder characterised by chronic abdominal pain, discomfort, bloating and alteration of bowel habits in the absence of any detectable organic cause.

531 J Graves' disease is caused by autoantibodies to the TSH receptor that activate it, thereby stimulating thyroid hormone synthesis and secretion, and thyroid growth.

532 C Subacute thyroiditis is a self-limiting, virally induced inflammation of the thyroid characterised by a febrile illness and swelling of the thyroid, with subsequent damage to the thyroid tissue causing leakage of thyroid hormones into the circulation.

533 F T_3 resin uptake (T_3RU) helps estimate the availability of thyroxin binding globulin (TBG). The higher the level of TBG, the lower the value of T_3 resin uptake and vice versa. Changes in thyroid function tests during pregnancy include a transient suppression of TSH and stimulation of triiodothyronine. Serum total T_4 and total T_3 steadily increase during pregnancy to approximately 1.5 times the non-pregnant level by mid second trimester. Whereas serum free T_4 and free T_3 gradually decrease during pregnancy.

534 G In T_3 resin uptake, lower than normal levels may be associated with hypothyroidism, acute hepatitis, pregnancy or use of oestrogen. Greater than normal levels may be associated with hyperthyroidism, renal failure, nephrotic syndrome or protein malnutrition.

535 A Non-toxic goitre refers to thyroid enlargement with a normal thyroid function.

536 H A deficiency in TBG is suspected when abnormally low serum total thyroid hormones concentrations are encountered in clinically euthyroid subjects in the presence of normal TSH.

537 B The limited cutaneous form of systemic sclerosis scleroderma is often referred to as CREST syndrome. CREST is an acronym for the five main features: **C**alcinosis, **R**aynaud's syndrome, o**E**sophageal dysmotility, **S**clerodactyly and **T**elangiectasia.

538 J Takayasu's arteritis is a form of large vessel granulomatous vasculitis. It typically affects young or middle-aged women of Asian descent (females : males = 9 : 1). It mainly affects the aorta and its branches, as well as the pulmonary arteries.

539 D Sjögren's syndrome can exist as a disorder in its own right (primary Sjögren's syndrome) or it may develop years after the onset of an associated rheumatic disorder, e.g. rheumatoid arthritis, systemic lupus erythematosus, scleroderma or primary biliary cirrhosis (secondary Sjögren's syndrome).

540 C The outlook for Reiter's syndrome is reasonably good, and most symptoms improve within 3–12 months. Occasionally, symptoms recur at some point in the future.

541 G PMR is a syndrome with pain or stiffness, usually in the neck, shoulders and hips, which is often worse in the morning. It may be caused by an inflammatory condition of blood vessels, but muscle biopsies are normal. It may be associated with temporal arteritis. It is usually treated with long courses of oral steroids. It usually resolves within 18 months after treatment.

542 L The hallmark result from laboratory tests that defines antiphospholipid syndrome (APS) is the presence of antiphospholipid antibodies. As cardiolipin is the dominant antigen used in most serologic tests for syphilis, these patients may have a false-positive test result for syphilis.

543 A Most patients with PDA present with a machinery murmur and are asymptomatic. Signs and symptoms of PDA are the result of left-to-right shunting and are proportional to the magnitude of the blood flow through the ductus.

544 G Coarctation of the aorta is best diagnosed clinically based on simultaneous palpation of femoral and brachial pulses. Blood pressure in both arms and one leg must be determined, as a pressure difference of more than 20 mmHg in favour of the arms may be considered evidence of coarctation of the aorta.

545 B ASD can go undiagnosed for decades due to subtle physical findings and a lack of symptoms. The findings on physical examination depend on the degree of left-to-right shunt.

546 E The clinical picture and functional impairment of VSDs primarily depend on the size of the defect, the status of the pulmonary vasculature and the degree of shunting, and less on the location of the VSD.

547 D Ebstein's anomaly is a congenital heart condition where there are abnormal attachments of the tricuspid valve leaflets to the annulus of the tricuspid valve. Examination is characterised by a gallop rhythm caused by widely split first and second heart sounds, as well as a third or fourth heart sound.

548 H In Fallot's tetralogy, cyanosis of the lips and nail bed is usually pronounced at birth. At the age of 3–6 months, the fingers and toes show clubbing.

549 A This is a case of tension pneumothorax resulting in lung collapse. An intercostal drain is the most definitive initial treatment of a tension pneumothorax.

550 E Widened mediastinum is a mediastinum wider than 8 cm on CXR. In the context of this case, it is vital to exclude a pericardial effusion or a cardiac temponade.

551 J This is a lung abscess. The fluid level is formed of pus. In the context of alcoholism, this is usually due to aspiration associated with impaired level of consciousness.

552 E In this clinical scenario, it is important to exclude cancer as a likely cause of those clinical features, and hence the need for a chest CT scan, which may later be followed by a bronchoscopy and biopsy.

553 A Necrotising granulomatous vasculitis may be associated with Wegener's granulomatosis, AIDS and cocaine abuse.

554 E Nodular glomerulosclerosis is the lesion of Kimmelstiel–Wilson disease, one of the forms of diabetic glomerulosclerosis.

555 D Focal segmental glomerulosclerosis may be primary or secondary to reflux nephropathy, Alport syndrome, heroin abuse or HIV. It presents as a nephrotic syndrome with varying degrees of impaired renal function.

556 C The WHO has divided lupus nephritis into five classes based on the biopsy:
- Class I is minimal mesangial glomerulonephritis.
- Class II is mesangial proliferative lupus nephritis.
- Class III is focal proliferative nephritis.
- Class IV is diffuse proliferative nephritis.
- Class V is membranous nephritis.

557 G Pre-eclampsia complicates approximately 5% of all pregnancies, making it the most common glomerular disease in the world. It is characterised by new-onset glomerular endotheliosis, which represents a specific variant of thrombotic microangiopathy.

558 B Goodpasture's syndrome describes the triad of diffuse pulmonary haemorrhage, glomerulonephritis, and circulating anti-glomerular basement membrane antibodies.

559 A β-blockers, together with ACE inhibitors, are vital in the management of cardiac failure. They are certainly indicated in this case, particularly in view of the relative tachycardia (in heart failure patients, the aim is for a pulse around 60 bpm).

560 B ACE inhibitors are indicated as a first line in such patients. It is good practice to exclude renal artery stenosis in young patients by requesting a renal ultrasound scan before starting treatment. If that is not possible, then treatment may be started provided renal function test is performed prior to and 1 week after starting ACE inhibitors.

561 G A 24-hour tape offers a good opportunity to diagnose the underlying cause of the problem. In many cases the cause may be atrial or ventricular ectopics, but more sinister rhythms, e.g. paroxysmal atrial fibrillation, may also be identified.

562 E Spironolactone is of benefit in class III and IV congestive cardiac failure, as demonstrated by the RALES trial. It is usually added as a third-line drug, after ACE inhibitors and β-blockers. Its use requires regular monitoring of renal function (particularly potassium levels).

563 I Young females presenting with palpitations must *always* have a thyroid function test prior to referral to a cardiac clinic, as thyrotoxicosis is frequently the underlying cause.

564 G Medullary thyroid carcinoma is associated with raised calcitonin and CEA.

565 E Raised AFP may be seen in testicular cancer, ovarian cancer, hepatoma, stomach cancer or pancreatic cancer.

566 D CEA is elevated in patients with colorectal carcinoma, gastric carcinoma, pancreatic carcinoma, lung carcinoma and breast carcinoma, as well as medullary thyroid carcinoma.

567 H Thyroglobulin is used as a tumour marker for well-differentiated papillary thyroid cancer.

568 J S-100 may be used as a tumour marker for melanomas, schwannomas, histiocytomas and clear cell sarcomas.

569 H Vertebral artery dissection is an increasingly recognised cause of stroke in patients younger than 45 years. An expanding haematoma in the vessel wall is the root lesion in vertebral artery dissection. This intramural haematoma can arise spontaneously or as a secondary result of minor trauma.

570 C Anterior spinal artery occlusion is also known as Beck's syndrome. It is usually associated with atherosclerosis of the aorta and may result from dissection of an aortic aneurysm. Clinical features include weakness and loss of pain and temperature sensation below the level of injury, with relative sparing of position and vibratory sensation.

571 E Multiple system atrophy is a degenerative neurological disorder. MSA is characterised by a combination of the following, which can be present in any combination:
- autonomic dysfunction
- Parkinsonism
- ataxia.

572 G Glioblastoma multiforme is the most common and most aggressive type of primary brain tumour. Symptoms depend on the location of the tumour rather than its pathological properties. The tumour can start producing symptoms quickly, but occasionally is an asymptomatic condition until it reaches an enormous size. Common symptoms include epilepsy, vomiting, headache and hemiparesis. The single most prevalent symptom is a progressive memory, personality or neurological deficit due to temporal and frontal lobe involvement.

573 D Alzheimer's is the most common form of dementia. In the early stages, the most commonly recognised symptom is the inability to acquire new memories, such as difficulty in recalling recently observed facts. When it is suspected, the diagnosis is usually confirmed with behavioural assessments and cognitive tests, often followed by a brain CT scan.

574 I Chronic inflammatory demyelinating polyneuropathy is characterised by progressive weakness and impaired sensory function in the legs and arms. Although it can occur at any age and in both genders, it is more common in young adults, and in men more than women. It often presents with tingling or distal numbness, weakness of the arms and legs, areflexia, fatigue, and abnormal sensations. It is closely related to Guillain–Barré syndrome and it is considered the chronic counterpart of that acute disease.

575 B Takayasu's arteritis should be suspected if there is one or more of the following signs: decreased radial pulse, difference in blood pressure between the two arms and/or hypertension. Most patients are treated with steroids and immunosuppressants. In some cases, angioplasty or stent placement may be needed.

576 D Kawasaki disease is a self-limiting febrile illness of childhood, characterised by vasculitis. It is of unknown aetiology. It may result in a spectrum of complications, ranging from asymptomatic coronary artery ectasis or aneurysm formation, giant coronary artery aneurysms with thrombosis to MI and sudden death.

577 H The terms 'giant cell arteritis' and 'temporal arteritis' are sometimes used interchangeably, because of the frequent involvement of the temporal artery. However, the pathology can involve other large vessels, e.g. the aorta. In 25% of cases, it may coexist with polymyalgia rheumatica. Examination reveals prominent temporal arteries and the temporal area may be tender. Fundal examination may reveal retinal ischaemic changes. Decreased pulses may be found throughout the body.

578 G The condition affects adults more frequently than children and males more frequently than females. It is more common in people with hepatitis B infection. P-ANCA is not associated with 'classic' polyarteritis nodosa, but is present in microscopic polyangiitis, which affects small vessels.

579 F Churg–Strauss syndrome (allergic granulomatous angiitis) is a rare syndrome affecting small- to medium-sized arteries and veins. It has three phases: allergic rhinitis and asthma; eosinophilic infiltrative disease, e.g. eosinophilic pneumonia or gastroenteritis; and systemic medium- and small-vessel vasculitis with granulomatous inflammation.

580 E Henoch–Schönlein purpura most commonly affects children, usually following an infection, e.g. pharyngitis. It causes palpable purpura, arthralgia and abdominal pain. When there is kidney involvement there may be haematuria and proteinuria.

581 C Ischaemic colitis occurs with greater frequency in the elderly, and is the most common form of bowel ischaemia. Mild to moderate cases are usually treated with IV fluids, analgesia and bowel rest until the symptoms resolve. Severe cases may require more aggressive interventions such as surgery and intensive care.

582 D Volvulus is a bowel obstruction in which a loop of bowel has abnormally twisted on itself. This results in ischaemia and intestinal obstruction. Acute volvulus therefore requires immediate surgical intervention to untwist the affected segment of bowel and possibly resect any unsalvageable portion. Volvulus occurs most frequently in middle-aged and elderly men.

583 F FMF is a hereditary inflammatory disorder caused by genetic mutations. The diagnosis is clinically made on the basis of the history of typical attacks, especially in patients from the ethnic groups in which FMF is more highly prevalent. During attacks, ESR, C-reactive protein and white blood cell count are elevated. A genetic test is also available that detects mutations in the *MEFV* gene.

584 A AIP is a rare autosomal dominant, metabolic disorder affecting the production of the haeme component of haemoglobin. AIP manifests itself by abdomen pain, neuropathies and constipation, but, unlike most types of porphyria, patients with AIP do not have a rash. Abdominal pain often is epigastric and colicky in nature, commonly with nausea and vomiting. Patients often are free of pain between attacks.

585 H PNH presents in any of the three syndromes or sets of symptoms:
- Haemolytic anaemia, which is usually in the form of intravascular haemolysis.
- Thrombosis involves the venous system, and it usually occurs in unusual veins, namely the hepatic, abdominal, cerebral and subdermal veins.
- Deficient haematopoiesis usually presents with anaemia despite the presence of an erythroid marrow with suboptimal reticulocytosis; in some cases, neutropenia and thrombocytopenia can occur in a hypoplastic bone marrow similar to aplastic anaemia.

586 J The majority of Meckel's diverticulum cases are asymptomatic. If symptoms do occur, they typically appear before the age of 2. The most common presenting symptom is painless rectal bleeding such as melaena-like black offensive stools, followed by intestinal obstruction, volvulus and intussusception. Occasionally, it may present with all the features of acute appendicitis. A memory aid is the rule of 2s: 2% (of the population); 2 ft (from the ileocaecal valve); 2 in (in length); 2% are symptomatic; 2 types of common ectopic tissue (gastric and pancreatic); *2* years is the most common age at clinical presentation; *2* times more boys are affected.

587 D Pernicious anaemia is a predisposing factor for gastric carcinoma.

588 G Nulliparity is a predisposing factor for ovarian cancer.

589 H Ulcerative colitis is a predisposing factor for colorectal cancer.

590 B Aniline dyes (which are no longer used in the developed world) predispose to urinary bladder carcinoma.

591 A Asbestosis predisposes to lung cancer.

592 F Epstein–Barr virus predisposes to Burkitt's lymphoma.

593 C The clue in this question is the raised haemoglobin, which is due to excessive secretion of erythropoietin.

594 A UTIs are more common in women than men, probably due to the shorter urethra. They can cause problems that range from dysuria to renal failure.

595 E The sclerotic areas in the spine refer to metastases from prostate cancer. Although bony metastases are usually blastic in nature, lytic lesions may occur, resulting in pathological fractures. Osteoporotic fractures due to prolonged LHRH therapy must be distinguished from pathological fractures.

596 B Smoking and cyclophosphamide are risk factors for bladder cancer. The presence of spinal metastases in this case makes a diagnosis of haemorrhagic cystitis unlikely (as it is also a possible complication of cyclophosphamide).

597 D Crystalluria is a clue to a diagnosis of renal stones in this case.

598 H The incidence of Edwards' syndrome (trisomy 18) increases with increasing maternal age.

599 E The incidence of Patau's syndrome (trisomy 13) increases with increasing maternal age.

600 G The incidence of double Y syndrome (47 XYY) is roughly one in 900 male births. This syndrome is characterised with a normal phenotype, tall stature and normal fertility. It is usually detected only during genetic analysis for another reason.

601 F The incidence of Klinefelter's syndrome (47 XXY) is roughly one in 1000 male births. The principal effects are the development of small testicles and reduced fertility.

602 D Down's syndrome (trisomy 21) is routinely screened during pregnancy by a nuchal ultrasound scan which is arranged between 11th and 13th week of gestation. If the result suggests high risk, then further investigation by amniocentesis may be required.

603 A Cases of Turner's syndrome where an X chromosome is completely missing are known as 'classical' Turner's syndrome. Cases where abnormalities only occur in the X chromosome of some of the body's cells are known as 'mosaic' Turner's syndrome, and they may display few or no symptoms.

604 B Hyponatraemia is the most common electrolyte disorder. It is usually due to fluid loss, e.g. vomiting and diarrhoea, or fluid accumulation, e.g. heart failure or SIADH.

605 D Hyperkalaemia is most commonly due to renal impairment and medications, e.g. ACE inhibitors, spironolactone, amiloride. Other causes include Addison's disease, hypoaldosteronism, haemolysis, burns, rhabdomyolisis and acidosis.

606 E In clinical practice, the most common cause of hypoglycaemia is iatrogenic, due to an overdose of insulin or oral hypoglycaemics.

607 A Hypokalaemia is mostly due to loss of potassium, e.g. diarrhoea and excessive sweating, medications (e.g. diuretics, insulin, salbutamol) and DKA. Other causes include alkalosis (as in vomiting), hypomagnesaemia and Conn's syndrome.

608 G Hypocalcaemia is usually due to vitamin D deficiency, hypoparathyroidism, renal impairment and alkalosis.

609 J Hypercalcaemia is usually due to hyperparathyroidism and malignancy. A useful mnemonic is: 'groans (constipation), moans (e.g. fatigue, lethargy and depression), bones (bone pain, especially if PTH is elevated), stones (kidney stones) and psychiatric overtones (including depression and confusion)'.

610 E Anaemia of chronic disease is a form of anaemia seen in chronic illness. It is likely to be resulting from production of hepcidin, which stops ferroportin from releasing iron stores.

611 G Aplastic anaemia is due to bone marrow failure, resulting in anaemia, thrombocytopenia and leucopenia, i.e. pancytopenia.

612 A This is due to erythropoietin production by hepatocellular carcinoma cells.

613 C In polycythaemia vera, the erythroid precursors do not require erythropoietin to avoid apoptosis.

614 F Erythropoietin is commonly used to treat anaemia in people with chronic kidney disease.

615 F SCID is a severe form of heritable immunodeficiency.

616 J Job's syndrome (hyperimmunoglobulin E syndrome) is a rare immune deficient disorder. Recurrent skin and lung infections and marked elevation of IgE levels are the hallmarks of hyperimmunoglobulin E syndrome.

617 H Patients with Chédiak–Steinbrinck–Higashi syndrome exhibit hypopigmentation of the skin, eyes and hair, prolonged bleeding times, easy bruisability, recurrent infections, abnormal natural killer cell function, and peripheral neuropathy.

618 A The mnemonic CATCH-22 can be used to describe DiGeorge syndrome, with the 22 to remind one that the chromosomal abnormality is found on chromosome 22:
  - **C**ardiac abnormality (especially tetralogy of Fallot)

- **A**bnormal facies
- **T**hymic aplasia
- **C**left palate
- **H**ypocalcaemia.

619 I Chronic granulomatous disease is an inherited disorder of phagocytic cells, resulting from an inability of phagocytes to produce bactericidal superoxide anions. This leads to recurrent life-threatening bacterial and fungal infections. The standard assay for phagocytic oxidase activity is the NBT test. The colourless compound NBT is reduced to blue by the activity of the phox enzyme system.

620 C Wiskott–Aldrich syndrome is a rare X-linked recessive disease characterised by eczema, thrombocytopenia, immune deficiency and bloody diarrhoea (secondary to thrombocytopenia).

621 D Down's syndrome can be diagnosed early in pregnancy (at about 15–16 weeks) by amniocentesis. There is a risk, however, of about one in 100–200 of a spontaneous miscarriage after the procedure. Accordingly, amniocentesis is only offered to women deemed to be at high risk of having a baby with Down's syndrome. Chorionic villous sampling usually takes place 10–12 weeks after the last period, earlier than amniocentesis. It is the preferred technique before 15 weeks.

622 B Intrahepatic cholestasis of pregnancy typically presents with troublesome itching. It usually occurs in the third trimester and resolves quickly after delivery. It is more common among twin and triplet pregnancies.

623 A A Kleihauer–Betke test, is usually performed on rhesus-negative mothers to determine the required dose of Rho(D) immune globulin to inhibit formation of Rh antibodies in the mother and prevent Rh disease in future Rh-positive children.

624 G All pregnant women with blood pressure greater than 140/90 mmHg with or without proteinuria should be referred to a day assessment or obstetric unit to exclude pre-eclampsia. A protein loss of over 300 mg in 24 hours is associated with an increased morbidity to the mother and her baby. In view of errors related to collection of a 24-hour urine sample, an elevated protein creatinine ratio of greater than 30 mg/mmol correlates with a 24-hour protein excretion greater than 300 mg and should be used to check for significant proteinuria.

625 F After 20 weeks, an S-F height measurement equal to the number of weeks of gestation +/– 2 cm can be considered normal. A reduced fundal height is likely to require an assessment involving CTG, AFI, Doppler and growth ultrasound.

626 B Pseudohypoparathyroidism is associated primarily with resistance to PTH. Patients have a low serum calcium and high phosphate, but PTH is actually appropriately high due to the hypocalcaemia.

627 K Osteomalacia is characterised by inadequate mineralisation of the bone secondary to inadequate amounts of available phosphorus and calcium. Osteomalacia in children is known as rickets, and because of this, use of the term 'osteomalacia' is often restricted to the milder, adult form of the disease.

628 L Multiple myeloma is associated with excessive tumour-induced, osteoclast-mediated bone destruction. Hypercalcaemia is the most frequent metabolic complication of myeloma in patients, and excessive osteolysis plays a major contributory role in its pathogenesis.

629 A Hypoparathyroidism can have a number of divergent causes: removal of or trauma to the parathyroid glands in thyroidectomy, autoimmune destruction, haemochromatosis, magnesium deficiency, DiGeorge syndrome and idiopathic.

630 D Primary hyperparathyroidism is usually due to an adenoma of the parathyroid glands (women : men = 3 : 1).

631 L Anorexia usually has its onset in adolescence and is most prevalent among adolescent girls. However, it can affect men and women of any age, race and socioeconomic and cultural background. It occurs in females 10 times more than in males.

632 A Those features are suggestive of thyrotoxicosis. All patients complaining of palpitations should have a thyroid function test.

633 H PCOS is one of the most common female endocrine disorders, affecting up to 10% of women of reproductive age, and is one of the leading causes of female subfertility. The syndrome acquired its most widely used name due to the common sign on ultrasound examination of multiple ovarian cysts. These 'cysts' are actually immature follicles, not cysts.

634 I Cryptomenorrhoea (haematocolpos) is a condition where menstruation occurs but is not visible due to an obstruction of the outflow tract, e.g. vaginal septum. It is surgically treated.

635 C Based on size, a prolactinoma can be classified as a microprolactinoma (< 10 mm diameter) or macroprolactinoma (> 10 mm diameter). It is commonly treated with bromocriptine or cabergoline.

636 E Large bowel obstruction can result from either mechanical interruption of the flow of intestinal contents or by the dilation of the colon in the absence of an anatomic lesion, i.e. pseudo-obstruction. Sigmoid diverticulitis and a perforated sigmoid secondary to carcinoma are clinically difficult to differentiate. Abdominal distention may be significant in patients with a large bowel obstruction. The caecum is the area most likely to perforate.

637 A Perforation usually results in classic findings of diffuse peritonitis with abdominal rigidity, guarding and rebound tenderness. Bowel sounds may initially be hyperactive but, with time, become absent. A diagnosis is made by taking an abdominal X-ray (seeking air under the diaphragm). Treatment generally requires immediate surgery.

638 D The leading cause of small bowel obstruction is post-operative adhesions (60%) followed by malignancy, Crohn's disease and hernias. Abdominal pain, often described as crampy and intermittent, is more prevalent in simple obstruction. Usually, pain that occurs for a shorter duration of time and is colicky and accompanied by bilious vomiting may be more proximal. Pain lasting several days, which is progressive in nature and with abdominal distension, may be typical of a more distal obstruction. Constipation is a late finding, as evidenced by the absence of flatus or bowel movements.

639 F Most people with diverticulosis do not have any discomfort but symptoms may include mild cramps, bloating and constipation. However, the most common symptom of diverticulitis is abdominal pain. The most common sign is tenderness around the left side of the lower abdomen.

640 K The history in this case suggests that the patient is an arteriopath and that results in a much higher risk of ischaemic colitis. The differential diagnosis in this case is ulcerative colitis, which is usually continuous from the rectum, with the rectum almost universally being involved. Colonoscopy shows erythema and friability of the mucosa, superficial ulceration which may be confluent, and pseudopolyps.

641 C Infectious colitis may be caused by *Campylobacter*, *Shigella*, *E. coli* or *Salmonella*. Patients with infectious colitis, in particular *Salmonella* and *Campylobacter*, are at increased risk of post-infectious irritable bowel syndrome and inflammatory bowel disease.

642 B Unlike ulcerative colitis, the inflammation of Crohn's disease is concentrated in some areas more than others, and involves layers of the bowel that are deeper than the superficial inner layers. Therefore, the affected segment(s) of bowel in Crohn's disease is often studded with deeper ulcers with normal lining between these ulcers. Skin involvement in Crohn's disease includes painful red raised spots on the legs (erythema nodosum) and an ulcerating skin around the ankles (pyoderma gangrenosum).

643 A The inflammation of ulcerative colitis tends to involve the superficial layers of the inner lining of the bowel. The inflammation also tends to be diffuse and uniform (all of the lining in the affected segment of the intestine is inflamed).

644 K Weight loss and rectal bleeding in an elderly male warrant urgent investigations to explore the possibility of colonic cancer.

645 F Painless rectal bleeding lining the stools is rather common in general practice, and is usually due to haemorrhoids.

646 E Tropicamide is an antimuscarinic drug that produces short-acting mydriasis and cycloplegia.

647 C Those are features suggestive of a seasonal allergic reaction, typically hay fever. Azelastine is a potent histamine-H_1-receptor antagonist.

648 H This is a case of herpes zoster ophthalmicus resulting in corneal ulcers. Fluorescein can detect foreign bodies in the eye, as well as damage to the cornea.

649 A Cupping of the optic disc is a sign of glaucoma. Timolol is used to treat open-angle and occasionally secondary glaucoma by reducing aqueous humour production through blockage of the β-receptors on the ciliary epithelium.

650 J This is a case of Sjögren's syndrome which should be treated with artificial tears, e.g. hypromellose.

651 B Those are classic features of cystitis.

652 H In post-streptococcal glomerulonephritis, the patient is usually male, aged 2–14 years, and suddenly develops puffiness of the eyelids and facial oedema in the setting of a post-streptococcal infection.

653 J There is evidence that some familial factors are involved in the development of benign recurrent haematuria and IgA nephropathy, which suggests that they may be closely related.

654 G Africans have the highest rates of Wilms' tumour (nephroblastoma). It is also more prevalent among females than males. Most instances of cancer occur among children under the age of five. Most nephroblastomas are unilateral.

655 A Purpura, arthritis and abdominal pain are known as the classic triad of Henoch–Schönlein purpura.

656 C *Molluscum contagiosum* is caused by a DNA poxvirus. It spreads through skin-to-skin contact. It is contagious until the lesions disappear, which if left untreated may be up to 6 months or longer. The incubation period can range up to 6 months, with an average between 2–7 weeks.

657 D CMV is one of the most common viral infections. It is estimated that around half of all adults in the UK have been infected by CMV. Most people develop the infection during early childhood or as teenagers. CMV causes few if any symptoms. It is only serious when it develops in immunocompromised patients, e.g. HIV-positive patients.

658 G Children of refugees are more likely to have missed their vaccinations. Infection with mumps usually gives a lifelong immunity.

659 I Parainfluenza viruses cause ~75% of the cases of croup. Repeated infection throughout the life of the host is not uncommon.

660 A Rotavirus is the most common cause of severe diarrhoea among infants and young children.

661 E The original description of Mallory–Weiss tear involves patients with persistent retching and vomiting following an alcoholic binge. However, Mallory–Weiss syndrome may occur after any event that provokes a sudden rise in intragastric pressure or gastric prolapse into the oesophagus.

662 A Acute gastritis can be broken down into two categories:
- erosive, e.g. superficial erosions, deep erosions, haemorrhagic erosions
- non-erosive, which is generally caused by *Helicobacter pylori*.

663 I Stomach cancer is often asymptomatic or causes only non-specific symptoms in its early stages. By the time symptoms occur, the cancer has often reached an advanced stage. The clue in this question is the sensation of fullness after small meals.

664 C Oesophageal varices are most often a consequence of portal hypertension, commonly due to cirrhosis. Schistosomiasis is readily treated using a single oral dose of praziquantel annually.

665 J Zollinger–Ellison syndrome is a triad of gastric acid hypersecretion, severe peptic ulceration and non-β-cell islet tumour of pancreas (gastrinoma). Patients with Zollinger–Ellison syndrome may experience abdominal pain and diarrhoea. The diagnosis is also suspected in patients without symptoms who have severe ulceration of the stomach and small bowel, especially if they fail to respond to treatment.

666 D Those are complications related to the oestrogen component of the COCP.

667 F The reversibility of sterilisation has very poor results, and that should be explained in counselling offered to couples prior to the procedure, whether vasectomy or tubal ligation.

668 A Periodic abstinence (rhythm method) entails not having sexual intercourse during the fertile period of the cycle (from 7 days before ovulation to 3 days after).

669 C Ectopic pregnancy risk is one in 20 if a woman becomes pregnant with IUCD in situ.

670 A The method is unreliable as the fertile period cannot be accurately calculated.

671 E Failure rates for coitus interruptus vary between 15%–28% per year.

672 D COCPs decrease the risk of ovarian cancer, endometrial cancer and colorectal cancer.

673 D COCPs can be used to treat polycystic ovary syndrome (PCOS), endometriosis, anaemia related to menstruation and dysmenorrhoea.

674 A Marcus Gunn pupil is observed during the swinging-flashlight test whereupon the patient's pupils constrict less (therefore appearing to dilate) when a bright light is swung from the unaffected eye to the affected eye. The affected eye still senses the light and produces pupillary sphincter constriction to some degree, albeit reduced. The most common cause of Marcus Gunn pupil is a lesion of the optic nerve proximal to the optic chiasma or severe retinal disease.

675 I Holmes–Adie pupil is a neurological disorder characterised by a tonically dilated pupil. It is caused by damage to the post-ganglionic fibers of the parasympathetic nerve fibres of the eye, usually by a viral or bacterial infection.

676 B Horner's syndrome is caused by damage to the sympathetic nervous system. Signs that are found in all patients on the affected side of the face include partial ptosis, slight elevation of the lower lid, anhidrosis and enophthalmos. Sometimes there is flushing on the affected side of the face. The pupil's light reflex is maintained as it is controlled via the parasympathetic nervous system.

677 H Argyll Robertson pupils are bilateral small pupils that constrict when the patient focuses on a near object, but do not constrict when exposed to bright light, i.e. they accommodate but do not react. They are a highly specific sign of neurosyphilis.

678 F This sign may be absent if other drugs are involved.

679 C A complete oculomotor nerve palsy results in a characteristic down and out position in the affected eye. The eye will be displaced downward because the superior oblique (innervated by the fourth cranial nerve) is unantagonised by the paralysed superior rectus and inferior oblique, and displaced outward because the lateral rectus (innervated by the sixth cranial nerve) is unantagonised by the paralysed medial rectus. Other features include ptosis and mydriasis.

680 J Therapeutic range for digoxin (for 6–12 hours post dose) is 1.0–2.6 nmol/L. However, toxicity may occur with a level of less than 1.3 nmol/L if there is hypokalaemia.

681 M While no specific monitoring tests are essential for ACE inhibitors, it is recommended to check the renal function prior to starting treatment and 1 week after any change in the dose, because of the risk of renal impairment and hyperkalaemia.

682 G Fluconazole may result in abnormal liver function tests.

683 A Amiodarone may result in abnormal thyroid function.

684 H HbA1c monitoring is the most commonly used method for assessing diabetes management.

685 D INR must be regularly checked in all patients on warfarin.

686 B Carbimazole may result in neutropenia.

687 E In patients on heparin, aPTT should be checked 4–6 hours after bolus dosage and every 24 hours thereafter.

688 L Unilateral vocal fold paralysis occurs from a dysfunction of the recurrent laryngeal or vagus nerve innervating the larynx. In this case, smoking and weight loss point towards bronchial carcinoma which probably infiltrated the left recurrent laryngeal nerve.

689 D Pharyngeal and laryngeal candidiasis may complicate long-term use of steroid inhalers.

690 K The clue in this question is the patient's occupation, which requires raising his voice. Typically, the nodules appear on the junction of the anterior and middle two-thirds of the vocal cord. The nodules appear as symmetrical swellings on both sides of the vocal cords.

691 H Most laryngeal cancers are squamous cell carcinomas and originate in the glottis. Supraglottic cancers are less common, and subglottic tumours are least frequent. Smoking is the most important risk factor for laryngeal cancer.

692 G Papillomas are benign epithelial tumours that are caused by infection with the human papilloma virus. They are the most common benign tumours affecting the larynx and upper respiratory tract. Malignant degeneration to squamous cell carcinoma may occur, but is very rare.

693 J Ortner's syndrome is a rare condition referring to recurrent laryngeal nerve palsy due to cardiovascular disease. The most common cause is a dilated left atrium due to mitral stenosis, but other causes including pulmonary hypertension, thoracic aortic aneurysms, and aberrant subclavian artery syndrome have been reported.

694 B At 2–5 months, a baby can glance at a rattle in hand and visually recognise its mother.

695 D At 7–10 months, a baby can feed itself a biscuit and transfer objects between hands.

696 G At 18–24 months, a baby can use a spoon and say more than 50 words.

697 H At 3 years, a child can ride a tricycle and sing a few nursery songs.

698 F At 14–18 months, a baby can point to a body part and run well.

699 E At 11–14 months, a baby can take two steps independently and release toys to others.

700 I At 4 years, a child can hop and count three to four objects.

701 C At 4–7 months, a baby can show displeasure over the loss of a toy and visually follow a dropped object.

702 J At 5 years, a child knows the days and counts to 10.

703 K At 6–8 years, a child prints words from memory and reads simple stories.

704 A Ramipril may cause birth defects or foetal death if given during pregnancy.

705 D Danazol is contraindicated in pregnancy and clinicians should give careful contraceptive advice to patients commencing or continuing danazol therapy in view of virilisation risk to female foetuses.

706 F Lithium appears to increase the risk of birth defects, especially heart defects. The risk is higher if lithium is taken during the first trimester of pregnancy.

707 L Misoprostol is commonly used for labour induction. It causes uterine contractions and effacement of the cervix.

708 G Aspirin is not recommended during the third trimester of pregnancy due to risk of closure of foetal ductus arteriosus and pulmonary hypertension.

709 B Cephalexin may be used in the management of severe infections during pregnancy.

710 E Dapsone is used in the treatment of leprosy and dermatitis herpetiformis. Neonatal hyperbilirubinaemia has been attributed to the use of dapsone during pregnancy.

711 C Grey baby syndrome is a rare but serious side effect that occurs in newborn infants (especially premature babies) following the intravenous administration of chloramphenicol.

712 E Bilateral lesions of the primary visual cortex may cause blindness. The cortically blind patient may have no vision but pupillary responses are intact and fundoscopy is normal.

713 A Those features are suggestive of acromegaly. The enlargement of the pituitary gland in the case of a macroadenoma results in compression of the optic chiasma, leading to bitemporal hemianopia.

714 J Amaurosis fugax is loss of vision in one eye due to a temporary lack of blood flow to the retina. It may be a sign of an impending stroke. It is a symptom of carotid artery disease. It occurs when a piece of plaque in a carotid artery breaks off and travels to the retinal artery. Visual loss usually only lasts seconds but may last several minutes.

715 L This is a case of multiple sclerosis. The first symptom of MS for around one in four people with MS is a disturbance of vision. Optic neuritis can cause pain behind the eye and visual loss that usually only affects one eye.

716 K Optic atrophy manifests as changes in the colour and the structure of the optic disc associated with variable degrees of visual dysfunction.

717 H Tensilon is the trade name for edrophonium chloride. The Tensilon test is an injection of edrophonium chloride used to diagnosis myasthenia gravis. Tensilon blocks the action of acetylcholinesterase, thus temporarily prolonging muscle stimulation. In a patient without MG, the Tensilon test will not produce an obvious increase in a previously weak muscle.

718 E The MCA is the largest cerebral artery and is the vessel most commonly affected by cerebrovascular accident. Main trunk occlusion on either side causes contralateral hemiplegia, eye deviation towards the side of the MCA infarct, contralateral hemianopia, and contralateral hemianaesthesia. Trunk occlusion involving the dominant hemisphere causes global aphasia.

719 C The motor and reflex changes secondary to thoracic cord compression depend on the level of the lesion:
- midthoracic – paralysis of intercostal muscles and upper motor neurone signs in the lower limbs.
- T9–T10 lesion – loss of abdominal reflexes, upward displacement of umbilicus and upper motor neurone signs in the lower limbs.
- T12–L1 lesion – loss of cremasteric reflex, normal abdominal reflexes and upper motor neurone signs in the lower limbs.

720 G Guillain–Barré syndrome is an acute inflammatory demyelinating polyneuropathy characterised by progressive symmetric ascending muscle weakness, paralysis and hyporeflexia with or without sensory or autonomic symptoms. It is believed to result from autoimmune humoral- and cell-mediated responses to a recent infection or other medical problems.

721 L Chronic alcoholic myopathy is a gradually evolving syndrome of proximal weakness and atrophy that complicates years of alcohol abuse. Typically, it is associated with a painless weakness affecting predominantly the hip and shoulder girdles, developing over weeks or months with significant muscle atrophy. However, acute muscle injury triggered by further alcohol binges may result in muscle pain.

722 I There are three main types of MND:
- Amyotrophic lateral sclerosis is the most common form of MND and accounts for 60%–70% of cases, who usually die within 2–5 years after the onset of symptoms.
- Progressive bulbar palsy accounts for 20% of cases, who usually die within 6 months to 3 years after the onset of symptoms.
- Progressive muscular atrophy accounts for 10% of cases, who usually die within 5–10 years after the onset of symptoms.

723 A Retinitis pigmentosa is a genetic progressive retinal dystrophy where night blindness precedes tunnel vision by many years.

724 D Argyll Robertson pupils are extremely uncommon in developed countries as syphilis is usually treated at a very early stage.

725 C In central retinal artery occlusion, the foveola assumes a cherry red spot because of a combination of two factors: the intact retinal pigment epithelium and choroid underlying the fovea, and the foveolar retina is nourished by the choriocapillaris.

726 B Bitemporal hemianopia is usually due to pituitary macroadenomas, craniopharyngiomas and meningiomas.

727 H Homonymous hemianopia can be congenital, but is usually caused by a CVA, trauma, tumours, infection or after a surgical procedure.

728 K Fuchs' heterochromic iridocyclitis is a condition characterised by a low-grade, asymptomatic uveitis in which the iris in the affected eye becomes hypochromic.

729 F Angioid streaks (Knapp streaks) are small breaks in Bruch's membrane in the retina. They are often associated with pseudoxanthoma elasticum, but are also noted in conjunction with Paget's disease, sickle cell anaemia and Ehlers–Danlos syndrome.

730 L In Graves' disease, the displacement of the eye is due to abnormal connective tissue deposition in the orbit and extraocular muscles which can be confirmed by an MRI scan.

731 G Bulbar palsy is characterised by bilateral impairment of function of the cranial nerves V, VII, IX, X and XI, which occurs due to lower motor neurone lesion either at nuclear or fascicular level in the medulla oblongata or from bilateral lesions of the lower cranial nerves outside the brainstem.

732 L Dysphagia to solids should always be investigated to exclude oesophageal carcinoma.

733 I GORD may lead to Barrett's oesophagus, which predisposes to carcinoma. Due to the risk of progression to Barrett's, oesophagogastroduodenoscopy (OGD) every 5 years is recommended for patients with chronic GORD.

734 K Cardiac achalasia is usually diagnosed by oesophageal manometry and barium swallow. Treatment options include sublingual nifedipine, botulinum toxin and dilation in those who fail medical management or surgical myotomy, though none of those options offers a cure.

735 A Oesophageal candidiasis occurs in immunocompromised patients. The diagnosis can be easily made with an oesophagogastroduodenoscopy (OGD). The current first-line treatment is a single dose of fluconazole (750 mg).

736 D Agoraphobia is an anxiety disorder defined as a fear of open spaces, crowds or uncontrolled social conditions. It is treated by cognitive behavioural therapy, SSRIs and benzodiazepines.

737 A PTSD occurs in up to 30% of people who experience traumatic events. It affects around 5% of men and 10% of women at some point during their lives, and can occur at any age, including during childhood. Approximately 40% of people with PTSD develop the condition after someone close to them suddenly dies.

738 F Paranoid schizophrenia sufferers are very suspicious of others and often have grand schemes of persecution at the root of their behaviour. Hallucinations, and more frequently delusions, are a prominent and a common part of the illness. It is the most common type of schizophrenia.

739 K CFS is defined by persistent fatigue unrelated to exertion, not substantially relieved by rest and accompanied by other specific symptoms for a minimum of 6 months. The disorder may also be referred to as myalgic encephalomyelitis (ME). The cause of CFS is currently unknown and there is no diagnostic laboratory test or biomarker.

740 L Delirium is an acute confusional state characterised by changes in arousal, perception deficit, altered sleep-wake cycle, and psychotic features such as hallucinations and delusions. It is often caused by a pathology outside the brain, such as infection or drug effects.

741 F Risk factors for ventricular tachycardia include myocardial infarction, structural heart disease or a family history of premature sudden death.

742 H Ventricular extrasystoles are a common finding in middle age, with patients noting an occasional missed beat. Patients with no ischaemic heart disease or cardiomyopathy have an excellent prognosis. However, ventricular extrasystoles post-myocardial infarction are associated with increased mortality.

743 D Risk factors for atrial flutter include long-standing hypertension, valvular heart disease, left ventricular hypertrophy, coronary artery disease, pericarditis, pulmonary embolism, hyperthyroidism and diabetes. Additionally, heart failure for any reason is a noted contributor to this disorder.

744 G Patients with Wolff–Parkinson–White syndrome may present with anything from mild chest discomfort or palpitations with or without syncope to severe cardiopulmonary compromise or cardiac arrest.

745 B In patients with structurally normal hearts, atrial tachycardia is associated with a low mortality rate. Patients with underlying structural heart disease, congenital heart disease or lung disease are less likely to be able to tolerate atrial tachycardia.

746 C Atrial fibrillation is the most common cardiac arrhythmia. It is often asymptomatic. Management is directed towards anticoagulation, rhythm control or rate control.

747 I Isolated first-degree heart block is asymptomatic and has no direct clinical consequences.

748 E Sinus tachycardia is usually a response to normal physiological situations, such as exercise and an increased sympathetic tone.

749 G The clue in this case is macrocytosis.

750 I β-thalassaemia minor is usually asymptomatic. It is characterised by mild anaemia with significant microcytosis which is disproportionate to the haemoglobin level. Iron levels are usually normal or elevated, though iron deficiency may also occur with β-thalassaemia minor.

751 D The median age at diagnosis of a myelodysplasia is between 60–75 years; a few patients are younger than 50. Males are slightly more commonly affected than females. It is characterised by anaemia, neutropenia and thrombocytopenia.

752 B Anaemia of chronic disease is characterised by normal or elevated ferritin, with reduced serum iron and TIBC.

753 E The clue in this case is that the patient is epileptic. Epileptic patients on phenytoin, phenobarbital or carbamazepine may suffer from folate deficiency due to reduced absorption.

754 H CLL is a disease of adults, but it can occur in teenagers, though rarely. Most newly diagnosed cases are men over the age of 50. Most cases are asymptomatic, being diagnosed by a routine blood test.

755 F Septic arthritis requires urgent treatment as it can destroy the joint within a few days. It should be considered whenever a patient presents with acute joint pain. The diagnosis of septic arthritis can be difficult as no test is able to completely exclude it.

756 D Gout mostly affects the metatarsal-phalangeal joint at the base of the big toe, accounting for half of cases. The heels, knees, wrists and fingers may also be affected. Renal underexcretion of uric acid is the primary cause of hyperuricaemia in about 90% of cases, while overproduction is the cause in less than 10%.

757 G Charcot joint (neuropathic osteoarthropathy) refers to progressive degeneration of a weight-bearing joint, a process marked by bone destruction, resorption and eventual deformity. It can result from any condition resulting in decreased peripheral sensation, proprioception, and fine motor control, e.g. DM, alcoholic neuropathy and cerebral palsy.

758 E Pseudogout is inflammation caused by calcium pyrophosphate crystals. Though it may be clinically indistinguishable from gout, it is suggested when abnormal calcifications (chondrocalcinosis) are seen in the joint cartilage on X-ray testing. Treatment of the acute phase of pseudogout is identical to that of gout. However, there is no specific treatment for the underlying cause of pseudogout, and no known prophylactic therapy exists.

759 L Reiter's syndrome is usually treated with NSAIDs, steroids and/or immunosuppressants.

760 D Vitamin D deficiency results in rickets in children and osteomalacia in adults (if vitamin D deficiency occurs after closure of the epiphyses). In the UK, the prevalence of vitamin D deficiency in all adults is around 14.5%, and may be more than 30% in those over 65 years old, and as high as 94% in otherwise healthy South Asian adults.

761 K Vitamin K deficiency may be due to reduced absorption (e.g. in bile duct obstruction), by intake of vitamin K antagonists or, rarely, due to nutritional vitamin K deficiency.

762 G Beriberi is due to due to vitamin B_1 deficiency. There are two major types of beriberi:
- wet beriberi – affecting the cardiovascular system
- dry beriberi and Wernicke–Korsakoff syndrome – affecting the nervous system.

763 C Scurvy is now very rare in the UK.

764 H Riboflavin deficiency has profound effects on the metabolism of carbohydrates, fats and proteins. It may be associated with chronic alcoholism, sickle cell anaemia, chronic fatigue syndrome and cataracts. It has been found to be a risk factor for the development of pre-eclampsia in pregnant women.

765 B Pellagra is most commonly caused by a chronic lack of niacin in the diet. Pellagra is classically described by 'the four Ds': diarrhoea, dermatitis, dementia and death. It is very rare in the UK.

766 J Vitamin B_{12} is stored in the liver, kidneys and other body tissues. As a result, vitamin B_{12} deficiency may not manifest itself until after 5 years of a dietary insufficiency. Vitamin B_{12} functions as a methyl donor and works with folic acid in the synthesis of DNA and red blood cells and is vitally important in maintaining the health of the myelin sheath.

767 B Cervical erosion (cervical ectropion) is a condition in which the endocervical columnar epithelium protrudes out through the external os of the cervix, undergoes squamous metaplasia and transforms to stratified squamous epithelium. It is a normal phenomenon, especially in ovulatory phase in younger women, pregnant women and those taking the combined oral contraceptive pill. Usually no treatment is indicated for clinically asymptomatic cervical ectropions.

768 D Ectopic pregnancy affects one in 100 pregnancies and can be easily confused with other causes of acute abdomen, e.g. appendicitis. If left untreated, about half of ectopic pregnancies will resolve without treatment (tubal abortions). The use of methotrexate has reduced the need for surgery. However, surgical intervention is still required in cases where the fallopian tube has ruptured or is in danger of doing so. This intervention may be laparoscopic or through a laparotomy.

769 F Hydatidiform (vesicular) mole may be complete or partial. Most complete moles are now diagnosed in the first trimester before the onset of the classic signs and symptoms (vaginal bleeding, hyperemesis and thyrotoxicosis). Patients with partial moles usually present with signs and symptoms consistent with an incomplete or missed abortion (vaginal bleeding and absent foetal heart sounds).

770 E Placenta praevia is the implantation of the placenta over or near the internal os of the cervix. It is a leading cause of vaginal bleeding in the second and third trimesters of pregnancy.

771 C In velamentous insertion, the umbilical cord inserts into the chorion laeve at a point away from the placental edge, and the vessels pass to the placenta across the surface of the membranes between the amnion and the chorion. One per cent of singletons have velamentous insertion, but it occurs in almost 15% of monochorionic twins and is common in triplets. Velamentous insertion can cause haemorrhage if the vessels are torn when the membranes are ruptured, most often with a vasa praevia.

772 E Examples of autosomal dominant disorders include Huntington's disease and neurofibromatosis-1.

773 H Examples of autosomal recessive disorders are cystic fibrosis, sickle cell disease and Tay–Sachs disease.

774 D Examples of X-linked dominant conditions include Rett syndrome, incontinentia pigmenti type 2 and Aicardi syndrome.

775 A Examples of X-linked recessive conditions include haemophilia A, Duchenne muscular dystrophy, Lesch–Nyhan syndrome, male pattern baldness and colour blindness.

776 I Since the Y chromosome is relatively small and contains very few genes, there are relatively few Y-linked disorders. The only known example of a Y-linked condition is hypertrichosis pinnae.

777 F The best known example of mitochondrial DNA inheritance is Leber's optic atrophy.

778 G Myotonic dystrophy is inherited in an autosomal dominant pattern with genetic anticipation (the symptoms of a genetic disorder become apparent at an earlier age as it is passed on to the next generation).

779 G Indications of forceps delivery:
- maternal – exhaustion, prolonged second stage, maternal illness, haemorrhage and drug-related analgesia
- foetal – foetal distress.

780 A Indications for CTG:

- maternal risks – pre-eclampsia, diabetes, antepartum haemorrhage, any significant maternal disease
- foetal risks – IUGR, prematurity, multiple pregnancy, breech presentation, meconium, premature rupture of membranes.

781 B An ultrasound would be useful to explore the cause of failure of engagement, e.g. placenta praevia or cephalopelvic disproportion.

782 F Foetal blood sampling is indicated in view of foetal distress.

783 H This is a case of severe foetal distress requiring an immediate Caesarean section.

784 C SSRIs are the most widely prescribed antidepressants in many countries. They increase the extracellular serotonin level by inhibiting its reuptake into the presynaptic cell. In addition to their use in clinical depression, SSRIs are frequently prescribed for anxiety disorders, panic attacks, obsessive–compulsive disorder, eating disorders, chronic pain and post-traumatic stress disorder. Other unlicensed uses include irritable bowel syndrome, lichen simplex chronicus and premature ejaculation.

785 D MAOIs are used as a last resort for treatment of depression in view of their significant side effects and interactions. They are also used for treating agoraphobia, Parkinson's disease (by targeting MAO-B enzyme), as well as providing an alternative for migraine prophylaxis.

786 F Mood stabilisers are used in management of bipolar disorders, borderline personality disorders and schizoaffective disorders. Many agents described as mood stabilisers are also classified as anticonvulsants, e.g. valproic acid, lamotrigine or carbamazepine.

787 A TCAs are one of the oldest classes of antidepressants and are still commonly used. Before the introduction of SSRIs, they were the standard treatment for depression. However, they are associated with more side effects than the SSRIs, and are now more likely to be reserved for cases when SSRIs are ineffective or inappropriate. They are also used in the management of neuropathic pain, ADHD, IBS, trichotillomania, nocturnal enuresis and Tourette's syndrome.

788 I Benzodiazepines enhance the effect of the gamma-aminobutyric acid (GABA), resulting in sedative, hypnotic, anxiolytic, anticonvulsant, muscle relaxant and amnesic action. Short-term use of benzodiazepines is relatively safe and effective, but long-term use is problematic due to tolerance, dependence and withdrawal syndrome on cessation of treatment.

789 B SNRIs are mainly used in the treatment of depression. They are also used in the treatment of anxiety disorders, obsessive–compulsive disorders, attention deficit hyperactivity disorder (ADHD), neuropathic pain and fibromyalgia. They act by increasing the levels of serotonin and noradrenaline in the brain.

790 G Typical antipsychotics are also known as first-generation antipsychotics or major tranquilisers. They are thought to act by blocking dopaminergic receptors, thereby interfering with dopaminergic transmission. There is growing evidence to suggest that typical antipsychotics also affect other neurotransmitter systems, e.g. cholinergic, α-adrenergic, histaminergic and serotonergic mechanisms. Typical antipsychotics are, therefore, essentially pharmacologically 'dirty' drugs and their use may consequently increase the risk of a wide variety of undesirable side effects.

791 E RIMAs selectively and reversibly inhibit monoamine oxidase A (MAO-A). They are safer than MAOIs. They are used in the treatment of depression and dysthymia, though they are rarely used due to their limited efficacy in comparison to other antidepressants.

792 H Atypical antipsychotics are also known as second-generation antipsychotics. They differ from typical antipsychotics in that they are less likely to cause extrapyramidal symptoms.

793 J In ABO haemolytic disease of the newborn, maternal IgG antibodies with specificity for the ABO blood group system pass through the placenta to the foetal circulation causing haemolysis, leading to foetal anaemia.

794 H Breast milk jaundice is characterised by indirect hyperbilirubinaemia in a breastfed baby that develops after the first 4–7 days of life, persists longer than physiologic jaundice and has no other identifiable cause. It should be differentiated from breastfeeding jaundice, which manifests in the first week of life and is caused by insufficient production or intake of breast milk.

795 G Biliary atresia is a congenital condition in which the biliary tree becomes progressively sclerosed and occluded. The main intrahepatic ducts become obliterated and death occurs in 98% of individuals by 2 years old.

796 F Up to half of the foetuses who become infected with toxoplasmosis during the pregnancy are born prematurely.

797 L Most infants develop visible jaundice due to elevation of unconjugated bilirubin concentration during their first week. Several possible mechanisms may be involved: increased bilirubin load, reduced hepatic uptake of bilirubin, reduced conjugation of bilirubin and defective bilirubin excretion.

798 E A wheal is an itchy, pale red papule or plaque that disappears within 24–48 hours. It is typically seen as a part of an allergic reaction.

799 J Onycholysis is the painless separation of the nail from the nail bed.

It can be associated with several conditions, e.g. psoriasis, lichen planus and atopic dermatitis.

800 B Perifollicular haemorrhage is characteristic of scurvy.

801 C Spider naevi are found only in the distribution of the superior vena cava. They are due to failure of the sphincteric muscle surrounding a cutaneous arteriole. The central red dot is the dilated arteriole and the red 'spider legs' are small veins carrying away the blood. If momentary pressure is applied, it is possible to see the emptied veins refilling from the centre. The dilation is caused by increased oestrogen levels in the blood as in pregnancy, hormonal contraception and liver cirrhosis.

802 A The characteristic diagnostic finding of alopecia areata is the exclamation-point hair which may be seen at the margin of the patch. These are broken, short hairs that taper at the base.

803 F Café au lait spots are seen with tuberous sclerosis, neurofibromatosis and Peutz–Jeghers syndrome, in addition to a few rare conditions.

804 L Erythema nodosum may be associated with:
- infections – streptococcal (most common), TB, syphilis, infectious mononucleosis and mycoplasma
- pregnancy
- iatrogenic sources – sulphonamides, penicillins and oral contraceptive pills
- autoimmune diseases and other conditions – ulcerative colitis, Behçet's disease and sarcoidosis
- malignancy – leukaemia and lymphoma.

805 D De Morgan's spots (cherry angiomas) are cherry red papules on the skin due to proliferation of capillaries. They are the most common kind of angioma. Their frequency increases with age. Rarely, they may be associated with a malignancy, and in that case they tend to appear suddenly.

806 J A branchial cleft cyst is an oval, mobile cystic mass that develops under the skin between the sternocleidomastoid and the pharynx. It is a remnant of embryonic development and results from a failure of obliteration of the branchial cleft. Most branchial cleft cysts are asymptomatic, but they may become infected.

807 C Classic features of lymphoma are fever, night sweats, weight loss and lymphadenopathy. TB may present with very similar features.

808 K The clue in this case is the history of heavy smoking, old age and the fact that the patient is male. All those factors point towards a malignancy, specifically laryngeal cancer, though lung cancer involving the left recurrent laryngeal nerve should also be suspected. Hoarseness of voice in a smoker requires an urgent referral to a specialist to exclude cancer. Neck swelling in this case is due to cervical lymphadenopathy.

809 H A pharyngeal pouch is a diverticulum of the pharyngeal mucosa through Killian's dehiscence (an area of weakness between the two parts of the inferior pharyngeal constrictor – the thyropharyngeus and the cricopharyngeus – at their posterior margin). The pouch probably arises as a result of a relative obstruction at the level of the cricopharyngeus. At first, it develops posteriorly but then it protrudes to one side, usually the left. As it enlarges, it displaces the oesophagus laterally. The diagnosis is confirmed by barium swallow. Endoscopy does not add further diagnostic information and may be dangerous because of the risks of perforation.

810 D A thyroglossal cyst is a fibrous cyst that forms from a persistent thyroglossal duct. It usually presents as an asymptomatic midline neck mass below the level of the hyoid bone. It moves during swallowing or on protrusion of the tongue because of its attachment to the tongue via the tract of thyroid descent. It is treated by surgical resection.

811 J The two antibiotics most commonly used in treatment of TB are isoniazid and rifampicin for 6 months plus pyrazinamide and ethambutol for the first 2 months.

812 E If a patient is allergic to penicillin, then erythromycin may be used. If it is suspected that cellulitis was caused by a skin wound exposed to contaminated water, then a combination of two different antibiotics is given: doxycycline or ciprofloxacin in combination with flucloxacillin or erythromycin.

813 G No reliable parenteral treatment for pseudomembranous colitis exists. Vancomycin is the most reliable treatment, while metronidazole is the cheapest option, making it the preferred first-line antibiotic.

814 B Various regimes may be used in the management of hospital-acquired pneumonia depending on local guidelines. Other options include ceftazidime plus tobramycin or ticarcillin-clavulanic acid plus tobramycin.

815 A Trimethoprim is probably the most commonly used antibiotic for treatment of urinary tract infections in general practice.

816 D Various regimes are available for the management of community-acquired pneumonia depending on clinical features, suspected organism, age and whether the patient is hospitalised or treated in the community. Other options include azithromycin, levofloxacin or cefotaxime.

817 H The primary treatment for osteomyelitis is parenteral antibiotics that penetrate bone and joint cavities. Treatment is required for at least 4–6 weeks. After intravenous antibiotics are initiated on an inpatient basis, therapy may be continued with intravenous or oral antibiotics, depending on the type and location of the infection, on an outpatient basis. Other treatment combinations include a penicillinase-resistant penicillin, and a third-generation cephalosporin or clindamycin, and a third-generation cephalosporin.

818 C Azithromycin or doxycycline are recommended for the treatment of uncomplicated genito-urinary chlamydial infection. Amoxicillin is recommended for the treatment of chlamydial infection in pregnant women.

819 E Patau's syndrome (trisomy 13) is the least common and most severe of the viable autosomal trisomies. Median survival is less than 3 days.

820 D Klinefelter's syndrome is the most common sex chromosome disorder in males. Affected males are almost always infertile.

821 A Edwards' syndrome (trisomy 18) is the second most common autosomal trisomy, after Down's Syndrome, that carries to term.

822 C Down's syndrome may be associated with a congenital ventricular septal defect that can manifest as a pansystolic murmur.

823 B Incidence of Turner's syndrome is 1 : 2000. It may be diagnosed by amniocentesis or foetal ultrasound scan during pregnancy.

824 D Although the PID infection itself may be cured, effects of the infection may be permanent, thus highlighting the need for early diagnosis and start of antibiotic treatment.

825 G Fibroids are the most common benign tumours in females. Symptoms caused by uterine fibroids are a very frequent indication for hysterectomy.

826 A The definition of menorrhagia is a blood loss of greater than 80 ml or lasting longer than 7 days. A normal menstrual cycle is 25–35 days in duration, with bleeding lasting an average of 5 days and total blood flow between 25 and 80 mL.

827 E Transvaginal ultrasound is the most cost effective investigation for suspected adenomyosis, where it will show an enlarged uterus with a heterogeneous texture, without the focal well-defined masses that characterise uterine fibroids.

828 J Endometrial carcinoma is the most common female genital cancer. As approximately 75% of women with endometrial cancer are postmenopausal, the most common symptom is postmenopausal bleeding. However, diagnosis may be missed in perimenopausal females unless bleeding is heavy or frequent.

829 A Most experts believe that the risk of sexual transmission of HCV is low. Most studies show that only up to 3% of contacts contract

HCV through unprotected heterosexual intercourse with a long-term, monogamous HCV-positive partner.

830 F COCP is ideal for management of irregular heavy periods in non-smoking females below the age of 35.

831 D Large uterine fibroids may distort the uterine cavity, rendering it unsuitable for an IUCD.

832 D Depo-Provera is a very effective contraceptive. It is injected every 12 weeks. The most common side effects are menstrual spotting and/or amenorrhoea.

833 G The most commonly used post-coital contraception in the UK is Levonelle 1500 mg (single dose). It is most effective within the first 24 hours, but is still effective up to 36 hours post intercourse. In 2010, a new pill was introduced (EllaOne), which is effective up to 5 days post intercourse.

834 C In this case, the history of breast cancer excludes hormonal contraception.

835 D The clues in this case are the positive family history, hypertension and bilateral loin masses.

836 C Ureteric stones < 6mm in diameter may pass spontaneously. Ureteroscopy has become increasingly popular. A ureteroscope uses a laser to destroy or fragment encountered stones. Extracorporeal shock wave lithotripsy (ESWL) is still commonly used for stones < 10mm in diameter, as it is the least invasive form of intervention. However, some studies retrospectively linked (ESWL) to diabetes and hypertension.

837 J Aniline dye exposure is a well-known risk factor for urinary bladder carcinoma.

838 G A left renal cell carcinoma can cause left varicocele through obstruction of the left renal vein which drains the left testicular vein. This typically does not occur on the right as the right gonadal vein drains directly into the inferior vena cava.

839 I Lower back pain associated with symptoms of prostatism should always raise suspicion of metastatic prostatic carcinoma.

840 H Fever, haematuria and loin swelling in a young child require urgent assessment to exclude Wilms' tumour (nephroblastoma).

841 H *Streptococcus pneumoniae* (pneumococcus) is Gram-positive, alpha-haemolytic, anaerobic member of the genus *Streptococcus*. It can also cause sinusitis, meningitis, endocarditis, osteomyelitis and septic arthritis.

842 G *Campylobacter jejuni* is a species of curved, helical-shaped, non-spore forming, Gram-negative, microaerophilic bacteria. It is commonly associated with poultry, and it naturally colonises the digestive tract of many bird species. Infection with *C. jejuni* usually results in enteritis with symptoms lasting 1–7 days.

843 A *Neisseria meningitidis* is a Gram-negative, diplococcal bacterium. It exists as normal flora in the nasopharynx of 5%–15% of adults. Meningococci spread from person to person by airborne droplets of infected nasopharyngeal secretions.

844 F *Escherichia coli* is a Gram-negative, rod-shaped bacterium. Most *E. coli* strains are harmless, but some (e.g. serotype O157:H7) can cause serious food poisoning in humans. The harmless strains are part of the normal flora of the gut, and can benefit their hosts by producing vitamin K and by preventing the establishment of pathogenic bacteria within the intestine.

845 D *Staphylococcus aureus* is a facultative anaerobic, Gram-positive coccus, and is the most common cause of staph infections. It is frequently part of the skin flora found in the nose and on skin. About 20% of the human population are long-term carriers of *S. aureus*.

846 L *Clostridium difficile* is a species of Gram-positive, anaerobic, spore-forming bacilli of the genus *Clostridium*.

847 I Carcinoma of the base of the tongue may cause referred otalgia via the glossopharyngeal nerve.

848 D Carcinoma of the ear canal is rare and is most likely to be a squamous cell carcinoma. The most frequently observed symptoms are discharge from the ear canal, often tinged with blood, and hearing loss.

849 L Spondylotic changes are often observed in the ageing population. However, only a small percentage of patients with radiographic evidence of cervical spondylosis are symptomatic.

850 G Acute otitis media is most often purely viral and self-limited, as it usually accompanies viral upper respiratory infection. If the middle ear, which is normally sterile, becomes contaminated with bacteria, pus and pressure in the middle ear can result, and this is called acute bacterial otitis media. Viral acute otitis media can lead to bacterial otitis media in a very short time, especially in children, but it usually does not.

851 B Ramsay Hunt syndrome (herpes zoster oticus) is defined as an acute peripheral facial neuropathy associated with erythematous vesicular rash of the skin of the ear canal, auricle and/or mucous membrane of the oropharynx.

852 L The clue in this question is her GCSE exams, implying significant stress. Stress can interfere with hypothalamic function resulting in amenorrhoea.

853 F Women who use an IUCD are 3.5 times more likely to develop PID, especially during the first 4 months after insertion. Some studies indicate that the increased risk exists only in women who are also at risk for STDs (e.g. women who have multiple partners). Several studies suggest that IUCDs can be used safely in monogamous relationships.

854 B An inevitable miscarriage refers to the presence of an open cervix in the context of bleeding in the first trimester of pregnancy.

855 H Ovarian torsion usually occurs unilaterally in a pathologically enlarged ovary. Malignant tumours are much less likely to result in torsion than benign tumours. This is due to the presence of adhesions that fix the ovary to surrounding tissues.

856 A An ectopic pregnancy occurs in about one in 100 pregnancies. Risk factors include: pelvic inflammatory disease, infertility, use of an intrauterine device (IUCD), previous tubal or intrauterine surgery (e.g. D&C), smoking, previous ectopic pregnancy and tubal ligation.

857 I Eighty to ninety per cent of malaria cases in Africa are caused by *Plasmodium falciparum*. *P. falciparum* causes severe malaria via a distinctive property not shared by any other human malaria, that of sequestration. Within the 48-hour asexual blood stage cycle, the mature forms change the surface properties of infected red blood cells causing them to stick to blood vessels (a process called cytoadherence). This leads to obstruction of the microcirculation and results in dysfunction of multiple organs, typically the brain in cerebral malaria. Haemoglobinuria with renal failure may also occur.

858 F Diagnosis of *Schistosoma mansoni* infection is confirmed by the identification of eggs in stools. *Schistosoma haematobium* is associated with urinary schistosomiasis.

859 A Oesophageal candidiasis is an AIDS-defining condition, generally occurring in individuals with CD4 counts of < 100 cells/μL. It is the most common cause of oesophageal infection in persons with AIDS.

860 D Amoebiasis symptoms can range from mild diarrhoea to dysentery with blood and mucous in the stools (due to amoebae invading the lining of the intestine). Microscopy is still by far the most widespread method of diagnosis around the world. Inside humans *Entamoeba histolytica* lives and multiplies as a trophozoite. In order to infect other humans they encyst and exit the body. Another human can get infected by ingesting the cysts from contact with contaminated water, food or hands. If the cysts survive the acidic stomach, they transform back into trophozoites in the small intestine. Trophozoites migrate to the large intestine where they live and multiply. Both cysts and trophozoites are sometimes present in the faeces. Cysts are usually found in firm stool, whereas trophozoites are found in loose stool. Only cysts can survive longer periods (up to many weeks outside the host) and infect other humans. If trophozoites are ingested, they are killed by the gastric acid of the stomach.

861 K *Pneumocystis jirovecii* pneumonia is a fungal infection of the lungs, which used to be called *Pneumocystis carinii*. This fungus is common in the environment and does not cause illness in healthy people. However, it can cause a lung infection in immunocompromised people due to cancer, chronic use of corticosteroids or immunosuppressants, HIV/AIDS, or organ or bone marrow transplant. *Pneumocystis* pneumonia in those with AIDS usually develops slowly over days to weeks or even months, and is less severe. People with *Pneumocystis* pneumonia who do not have AIDS usually get sick faster and are more acutely ill.

862 G Toxoplasmosis is transmitted via exposure to infected raw meat or cat faeces. Toxoplasmosis cannot be passed on through person-to-person contact, but it can be passed from a pregnant woman to her unborn baby. In most cases, toxoplasmosis may be asymptotic due to good immunity. Up to half of the UK population will have a toxoplasmosis infection at some point in their lives. Once infected, a person is then immune from further infection for life. Diagnosis can be reached using polymerase chain reaction (PCR) to detect toxoplasma in blood.

863 K A simple faint is rather common in general practice. There is no reason for concern provided there are known provocative factors with associated prodromal symptoms which are unlikely to occur whilst sitting or lying.

864 I Following angioplasty +/− stent, driving must cease for 1 week. DVLA need not be notified.

865 A Visual acuity and field restrictions must be met in cases of night blindness.

866 J Following a CABG, driving must cease for 4 weeks. Driving may recommence thereafter provided there are no other disqualifying conditions.

867 B Following a CVA or TIA, driving must cease for 1 month. DVLA need not be notified unless there is a residual neurological deficit.

868 K Hypertensive patients may continue to drive without informing the DVLA unless treatment causes unacceptable side effects.

869 M First unprovoked epileptic seizure requires immediate cessation of driving for a minimum of 6 months.

870 G Patients suffering from Parkinson's disease may be licensed provided they pass medical examination. They are usually given short-term (1–3 years) licences.

871 K Patients suffering from migraine may continue to drive without informing the DVLA.

872 I Following a pacemaker implant, driving must cease for a minimum of 1 week. DVLA need not be notified.

873 K A post-traumatic scrotal haematocele requires urgent assessment by an ultrasound and/or surgical exploration to exclude testicular torsion or rupture, evacuate the haematocele and prevent the need for later orchidectomy.

874 L A hydrocele is caused by accumulation of clear fluid in the tunica vaginalis. Most hydroceles are benign and can be left untreated (primary hydrocele). However, a small proportion are due to testicular pathology, e.g. malignancy (secondary hydrocele).

875 A Testicular torsion is more common in the winter and in case of a large testis. The diagnosis is often made clinically, but if in doubt, an ultrasound is helpful to confirm or exclude the diagnosis. Emergency diagnosis and treatment is required in order to save the testicular viability. Clinically, epididymitis may be indistinguishable from testicular torsion.

876 H Acute epididymo-orchitis mostly occurs in young males. Organisms may reach the epididymis by retrograde spread from the prostatic urethra and seminal vesicles, or less commonly through the blood stream. Predisposing factors include urinary tract infection, urethral instrumentation and sexually transmitted infection. *E. coli* and *Chlamydia* in patients with a history of urethral discharge are the organisms most frequently cultured. Clinically, epididymo-orchitis may be indistinguishable from testicular torsion.

877 F The vast majority of teratomas secrete HCG and/or α-feto protein which can be measured in the serum and used as a tumour marker. They are less radiosensitive than seminomas.

878 E Seminoma originates in the germinal epithelium of the seminiferous tubules. It is one of the most curable cancers, with survival > 95% in the early stages. Treatment usually requires testicular excision. Placental alkaline phosphatase (PLAP) is raised in 50% of cases. HCG may also be elevated, but α-feto protein is normal.

879 A Primary hyperparathyroidism causes hypercalcaemia through the excessive secretion of PTH, usually by a parathyroid adenoma. It is almost three times as common in women as men.

880 F Pseudohypoparathyroidism is associated with PTH resistance. It is classified into types 1a, 1b and 2. Type 1a is characterised by short fourth and fifth metacarpals and a rounded facies. While biochemically similar, type 1 and 2 disease may be distinguished by the differing urinary excretion of cyclic AMP in response to exogenous PTH.

881 D Paget's disease is characterised by normal serum calcium, phosphorus and parathyroid hormone levels. However, in the setting of immobilisation, hypercalcaemia may ensue. ALP is typically raised.

882 C Tertiary hyperparathyroidism is a state of excessive secretion of parathyroid hormone after long-standing secondary hyperparathyroidism and resulting in hypercalcaemia. Tertiary hyperparathyroidism is commonly used at present in the context of persistent secondary hyperparathyroidism following successful renal transplantation.

883 G Pseudopseudohypoparathyroidism is a condition where the patient has the phenotypic appearance of pseudohypoparathyroidism type 1a but is biochemically normal. It is sometimes considered a variant of Albright hereditary osteodystrophy.

884 B Secondary hyperparathyroidism is the overproduction of parathyroid hormone secondary to a chronic abnormal stimulus for its production, usually due to chronic renal failure. Another common cause is vitamin D deficiency.

885 D This clinical scenario is suggestive of an ectopic pregnancy, with acute appendicitis as a less likely possibility. The simplest and most available test at a GP surgery is a pregnancy test. Such a patient would require an urgent assessment at the local A&E department, where she would typically have an ultrasound scan.

886 H Postmenopausal bleeding requires urgent assessment to exclude endometrial carcinoma. Tamoxifen is a risk factor for endometrial carcinoma. Transvaginal ultrasound is a useful tool for screening women with postmenopausal bleeding. Several studies have shown that demonstration of a normal endometrium virtually excludes the presence of endometrial carcinoma. This is important because 80%–90% of patients with postmenopausal bleeding do not have endometrial carcinoma.

887 K This woman is due for a cervical smear anyway. The NHS cervical screening programme in the UK offers screening to all women on a 3-yearly basis from the age of 25–49, then on a 5-yearly basis from the age of 50–64.

888 B This woman is perimenopausal. The diagnosis of menopause is confirmed by FSH levels > 40 IU/L.

889 M Breakthrough bleeding is an abnormal uterine bleeding occurring between periods, especially in women on combined oral contraceptives. In many cases, it may cease after one or two cycles. There is a higher risk among smokers.

890 B In gonorrhoea, the incubation period is 2–30 days, with most symptoms occurring between 4–6 days after being infected. Fifty per cent of women with gonorrhea are asymptomatic.

891 A Genital chlamydia is a sexually transmitted infection which is asymptomatic in up to 75% of women infected with the disease.

892 D Lymphogranuloma venereum (inguinale) is a sexually transmitted disease that primarily infects the lymphatics. The primary lesion of LGV occurs after an incubation period of 3–21 days following an exposure. The secondary stage of LGV occurs after a usual incubation period of 10–30 days (but it may be up to 6 months). This stage is characterised by the formation of enlarged, tender regional lymph nodes known as buboes. Tertiary LGV is characterised by proctocolitis.

893 I Typically, only women experience symptoms associated with *Trichomonas* infection. Symptoms include cervicitis, urethritis and vaginitis. It usually responds to metronidazole.

894 G Primary herpes simplex virus HSV-1 and HSV-2 infections are accompanied by systemic signs, longer duration of symptoms and higher rate of complications. Recurrent episodes are milder and shorter. Both HSV-1 and HSV-2 can cause similar genital and orofacial primary infections after contact with infectious secretions.

895 K Individual molluscum lesions may resolve spontaneously. They usually last 6 weeks to 3 months. However, the disease may propagate via autoinoculation, and so the outbreak may last from 6 months to 5 years.

896 G HONK is characterised by severe hyperglycaemia with marked serum hyperosmolarity, without evidence of significant ketosis. It can affect people of all ages, but is much more common in older type 2 diabetics.

897 A There are several clues in this case: hypernatraemia, hypokaemia and hypertension, which all point to Conn's syndrome.

898 K In this case, there are features suggestive of congestive cardiac failure with fluid overload (oedema, raised JVP, crackles). The history of hepatitis C and ascites suggests progression to cirrhosis. About 75%–85% of patients with ascites in the UK have cirrhosis. Normal creatinine levels exclude hepatorenal syndrome.

899 C Distal renal tubular acidosis (type 1 RTA) is caused by a renal defect causing failure to acidify the urine, resulting in acid accumulation in the blood. It is caused by amyloidosis, Fabry's disease, sickle cell disease, Sjögren's syndrome, systemic lupus erythematosus, Wilson's disease and certain drugs, e.g. lithium and amphotericin B. It is characterised by normal anion gap metabolic acidosis and hypokalaemia.

900 E Pyloric stenosis occurs in adults due to scarring from chronic peptic ulceration resulting in a narrow pylorus. Pyloric stenosis causes persistent vomiting resulting in metabolic alkalosis, hypokalaemia and hypochloraemia.

901 F There are several clues in this case: history of autoimmune diseases, abdominal pain, hyperpigmentation, hyponatraemia and hyperkalaemia.

902 E Nitrous oxide is commonly known as laughing gas. When nitrous oxide is inhaled as the only anaesthetic drug, it is normally administered as a mixture with 30% gas and 70% oxygen. In the UK, it is commonly used by ambulance crews as a rapid and highly effective analgesic gas.

903 A Paracetamol is the most commonly used analgesic in the UK. With the exception of overdosing, it is considered safe.

904 H There are several medications available to the treatment of post-herpetic neuralgia, e.g. amitryptiline, carbamazepine, gabapentin, lamotrigine and pregabalin.

905 B The history suggests a pathological spinal fracture, which would require maximum analgesia, e.g. diamorphine.

906 L The history suggests gout, precipitated by diuretics. The dose of colchicine in acute gout is 1 mg followed by 500 µg every 2–3 hours, up to a maximum of 6 mg.

907 K Acute pancreatitis requires significant analgesia. While pethidine has traditionally been favoured over morphine, there is no definitive human study to support the widespread belief that morphine exacerbates pancreatitis by stimulating the sphincter of Oddi to contract. Accordingly, morphine is the drug of choice in a significant proportion of centres.

908 G Diamorphine is used as standard in management of acute myocardial infarction.

909 G Diagnosis of shingles is usually on clinical grounds as the rash follows a dermatomal pattern.

910 A Tinea corporis is one of the most common dermatological problems in general practice. It may result from contact with infected humans, animals or inanimate objects. Humidity is an important risk factor.

911 C Meningococcal rash is often present, but its absence does not exclude the diagnosis of meningococcal meningitis. On suspicion of meningococcal meningitis, intravenous antibiotics should be started, pending results of lumbar puncture, as delay in treatment worsens the prognosis.

912 B Tinea versicolour is characterised by a rash on the trunk and proximal extremities. Hypopigmentation is common among patients with dark skin, while hyperpigmentation is common among patients with lighter skin.

913 D Dermatitis herpetiformis is an autoimmune blistering disorder associated with gluten-sensitive enteropathy. It is extremely pruritic, and the vesicles are often excoriated to erosions by the time of physical examination.

914 H Many viruses can cause a rash in addition to other symptoms such as fever and cough. Many of these rashes are 'non-specific'. Viral rash varies in shape and size, but it often appears as blotchy red spots.

915 L Stevens–Johnson syndrome is a life-threatening condition affecting the skin in which the epidermis separates from the dermis. It is thought to be a hypersensitivity complex affecting the skin and the mucous membranes. Although the majority of cases are idiopathic, the main class of known causes is medications, followed by infections and cancers.

916 C Behçet's disease is a rare, systemic vasculitis often presenting with mucous membrane ulceration, ocular, gastrointestinal, pulmonary, musculoskeletal and neurological symptoms. There is no specific pathological testing or technique available for the diagnosis of the disease. However, the International Study Group criteria for the disease are highly sensitive and specific, involving clinical criteria and a pathergy test with a specificity of 95%–100%.

917 E Herpes zoster is due to activation of latent varicella zoster virus in neurones, usually several years or even decades following an infection with chickenpox. Interestingly, herpes zoster in children is often painless. Antiviral medications, e.g. acyclovir or famcyclovir, can reduce the severity and duration of herpes zoster if started within 72 hours of the appearance of the characteristic rash.

918 G Historically, syphilis was more predominant among sailors. Primary syphilis is characterised by a single chancre, secondary syphilis is associated with a skin rash, latent syphilis is asymptomatic, while tertiary syphilis is associated with gummata. Congenital syphilis may occur during pregnancy or during the birth process. Most infants are born without symptoms.

919 H The exact cause of aphthous ulcers is unknown, but there are several predisposing factors, e.g. trauma, stress, insomnia, sudden weight loss, food allergies, cow milk allergy, immune system reactions, citrus fruits, deficiencies in vitamin B_{12}, iron and folic acid, nicorandil and chemotherapy.

920 B Crohn's disease typically affects the ileum and/or the colon, but it can affect any part of the digestive system. Mouth ulcers are commonly associated with Crohn's disease.

921 B IBS is a diagnosis of exclusion, as routine clinical tests yield no abnormalities.

922 G Symptoms and signs of ovarian cancer can be vague, which may explain delayed diagnosis, particularly as there are no routine screening tests for ovarian cancer. Weight loss associated with increased abdominal girth raise suspicion about the possibility of an abdominal malignancy.

923 I Ovarian torsion classically occurs unilaterally in a pathologically enlarged ovary. Approximately 60% of torsion occurs on the right side. A unilateral tender adnexal mass may be palpable. However, absence of such a finding does not exclude the diagnosis. Women undergoing induction of ovulation for infertility carry an even greater risk, as numerous theca lutein cysts significantly expand the ovarian volume.

924 D The raised tender lesions refer to erythema nodosum.

925 C Laparoscopy is the current criterion standard for the diagnosis of PID, as no single test is highly specific or sensitive for the disease. Risk factors for PID include multiple sexual partners, a history of prior STD, a history of sexual abuse, surgical procedures, e.g. endometrial biopsy, curettage, and hysteroscopy (as they break the cervical barrier), and younger age (due to increased cervical mucosal permeability, a larger zone of cervical ectopy, a lower prevalence of protective chlamydial antibodies and increased risk-taking behaviour).

926 L The diagnosis of diverticulitis can be made on clinical grounds, but a CT scan of the abdomen is considered the best imaging method to confirm the diagnosis. Contrast enema is not the imaging modality of choice during an acute episode and should only be considered in mild to moderate uncomplicated cases of diverticulitis when the diagnosis is in doubt. A water-soluble contrast should be used, as leakage of barium into the peritoneum would be catastrophic.

927 G Neuroleptic malignant syndrome is a combination of fever, rigidity and autonomic disturbance occurring as a complication of antipsychotic drugs.

928 H Guillain–Barré syndrome is an acute, inflammatory, post-infectious polyneuropathy. A typical presentation involves malaise with fever, vomiting, headache and limb pains followed by a progressive and ascending paralysis. This can lead to respiratory failure. Accordingly, it is considered a neurological emergency.

929 B Turner's syndrome may be suspected in pregnancy during an ultrasound. This can be confirmed by chorionic villous sampling or amniocentesis.

930 E Eaton–Lambert syndrome is a presynaptic myasthenic syndrome characterised by impaired release of acetycholine from nerve terminals. About 60% of patients have small cell lung carcinoma. The usual age of onset is between 50–60 years of age. Men are affected more than women.

931 C Treatment of Klinefelter's syndrome should address three major aspects of the disease: hypogonadism, gynaecomastia and psychosocial problems. Androgen therapy is the most important aspect of treatment. Men with Klinefelter's syndrome were considered infertile until the last decade, when artificial reproductive technologies (ART) allowed more than 50% of patients with Klinefelter's syndrome to have their own children through the combination of microsurgical testicular sperm extraction (TESE) and the use of freshly retrieved sperm for in-vitro fertilisation (IVF).

932 L Symptoms of Reiter's syndrome (reactive arthritis) typically appear within 1–3 weeks following a genito-urinary or a gastrointestinal infection.

933 F Antiphospholipid syndrome manifests clinically as recurrent venous or arterial thrombosis and/or miscarriage. Low-dose aspirin is commonly used in management. Hydroxychloroquine should be considered in patients with SLE.

934 G Patients with generalised tonic–clonic seizures do not have auras. An aura represents a simple partial seizure, and a reliable history of aura identifies the seizure as partial and not generalised. Within 10–20 minutes of a generalised tonic–clonic seizure, prolactin levels are elevated by five to 30 times the baseline values. An abnormality on CT scans is rare in patients with primary generalised tonic–clonic seizures. As CT will not detect most types of congenital structural brain abnormalities, MRI is the imaging modality of choice. The awake EEG of patients with generalised tonic–clonic seizure is often normal.

935 A Hyponatraemia is an occasional but serious complication of diuretic therapy. Virtually all cases of severe diuretic-induced hyponatraemia are due to a thiazide diuretic. A loop diuretic is much less likely to induce this problem. Another potential cause of hyponatraemia in patients with lung cancer is SIADH. Small cell cancer of the lung is the cause in 75% of cases of SIADH caused directly by a tumour. In some cases, the appearance of SIADH may be the first indication of a new diagnosis of cancer.

936 L Typical absence seizures are usually associated with generalised 3–4 Hz spike-and-slow-wave complexes on EEG. Typically, patients present with 'absence spells' lasting for a few seconds. Other symptoms such as behavioural problems may be the presenting complaint.

937 J A partial seizure with secondary generalisation starts in one limited area of the brain. The forms they take vary as much as other partial seizures. But then (sometimes so quickly that the partial seizure is hardly noticed), the seizure spreads throughout the brain, becoming generalised.

938 B One of the rare but serious complications of total thyroidectomy is tetany due to parathyroidectomy.

939 C Magnesium has a vasodilator effect on cerebral blood vessels. In hypomagnesaemia, cerebral vasospasm is believed to predispose to convulsions.

940 I Most subconjunctival haemorrhages are spontaneous. Precipitating factors include coughing, sneezing, straining or use of anticoagulants.

941 F Anterior uveitis is a common cause of a painful red eye. Management typically includes topical cycloplegics and corticosteroids.

942 A Keratitis caused by herpes simplex virus typically presents as a unilateral red eye with a variable degree of pain or ocular irritation. Photophobia and epiphora are common. However, vision may or may not be affected depending upon the location and extent of the corneal lesion.

943 H In closed-angle glaucoma, there is obstruction at the trabecular meshwork resulting in impairment of aqueous ouflow, leading to raised IOP. In this case, the significance of onset at the cinema is that darkness triggers pupillary dilatation, resulting in reduced aqueous outflow.

944 D Infective conjunctivitis is very common and is responsible for 35% of all eye-related problems recorded in GP surgeries in the UK. It is most common in children and the elderly.

945 L While trachoma is relatively common in certain parts of the world, Europe is now free of trachoma. Recurrent infections cause conjunctival scarring leading to trichiasis. Cobblestone appearance of the conjunctiva is characteristic of trachoma.

946 G A pterygium is a raised, triangular lesion composed of conjunctival tissue over the surface of the cornea. It usually occurs on the nasal side of the cornea and is often bilateral. Pterygia typically develop in individuals who have been living in hot dry climates due to long-term exposure to sunlight, especially during childhood and adolescence, and chronic irritation from the dry climate.

947 H Small cell lung cancer is different from other lung cancers in that it exhibits rapid growth, early spread to distant sites, significant sensitivity to chemotherapy and radiation, and frequent association with distinct paraneoplastic syndromes. Surgery usually plays no role in its management. Hypokalaemic alkalosis is seen in > 75% of patients with ectopic ACTH production.

948 J Thymoma is the most common neoplasm of the anterior mediastinum. No clear histological distinction between benign and malignant thymomas exists. The propensity of a thymoma to be malignant is determined by its invasiveness.

949 L Pleural mesothelioma is caused by asbestos exposure, which in this case is related to the patient's past employment.

950 D The most common feature of Hodgkin's lymphoma is asymptomatic lymphadenopathy (80% of patients). Constitutional symptoms (e.g. unexplained weight loss, fever, night sweats) are present in 40% of patients. Alcohol-induced pain at swollen lymph nodes is specific for Hodgkin's lymphoma and occurs in less than 10% of patients.

951 F Adenocarcinoma of the lung is a form of non-small cell lung cancer. Eighty per cent of lung cancers are non-small cell cancers, and of these, about 50% are adenocarcinomas. It begins in the outer parts of the lung, and can be present for a long time before it is diagnosed. It is the type of lung cancer most commonly seen in women and non-smokers.

952 E Squamous cell lung cancer is a form of non-small cell lung cancer. Eighty per cent of lung cancers are non-small cell lung cancers, and of these, about 30% are squamous cell lung cancer. It usually begins in the large airways in the central part of the lungs. Many patients have early symptoms, specifically haemoptysis. It often causes ectopic production of parathyroid hormone-related protein resulting in hypercalcaemia.

953 A Those are classic features of bacterial meningitis.

954 K The temporal artery should be biopsied if the diagnosis of GCA is in doubt, because the result would determine the appropriate treatment. Treatment should be started immediately, even if biopsy must be delayed. However, after starting systemic corticosteroids, biopsy becomes less useful. A positive biopsy confirms the diagnosis while a negative biopsy does not rule out GCA, since parts of the artery can be normal with 'skip lesions'. Biopsies of longer arterial section are more sensitive, and thus have better negative predictive values.

955 E Subarachnoid haemorrhage may be associated with subhyaloid haemorrhage and vitreous haemorrhage, which are visible on fundoscopy. This is known as Terson syndrome and is more common in more severe cases.

956 L About 70% of men and 85% of women develop a tension headache at some point during their lives. It can occur at any age, but most commonly begins during adolescence or young adulthood, with the highest frequency among those aged 20–50 years. Tension headache must have at least two of the following characteristics:
- pressing/tightening (non-pulsating) quality, located on both sides of the head
- mild or moderate intensity
- not aggravated by routine physical activity
- not associated with nausea or vomiting
- possible sensitivity to light or sound but not both.

957 H Cluster headache affects approximately 0.1% of the population, and men are more commonly affected than women. Cluster headaches are excruciating unilateral (though rarely bilateral) headaches of extreme intensity. The duration of an attack ranges from

15 minutes to 3 hours or more. The onset of an attack is rapid, and most often without the preliminary signs that are characteristic of a migraine.

958 D Idiopathic intracranial hypertension is characterised by increased intracranial pressure in the absence of a tumour or other diseases. It may occur in all age groups, but is most common in young obese women. It can be treated by a lumbar puncture (which can be diagnostic as well as therapeutic), acetazolamide (diamox) and as a last resort, surgically.

959 C Migraine is a common medical problem, affecting about 15% of adults in the UK. There are two types of migraine:
- classical (~30% of cases) – where there is an aura, e.g. visual problems (such as flashing lights), and stiffness in the neck, shoulders or limbs
- common (~70% of cases) – where there is no aura.

960 D Atrophic vaginitis is characterised by thinning and shrinking of urogenital tissues, as well as decreased lubrication due to the lack of oestrogen. It is a cause of post-coital and postmenopausal bleeding. It is usually managed by topical oestrogen.

961 B The most common symptoms caused by a foreign body in the vagina are bleeding or foul-smelling vaginal discharge. Less common symptoms may include pain or urinary discomfort.

962 K Miscarriage is very common, particularly in the first trimester. It is defined as the expulsion of an embryo or foetus due to accidental trauma or natural causes before approximately the 22nd week of gestation. A late, heavy, painful 'period' is often what is experienced in a mid-first trimester miscarriage and the cause is usually a chromosomal anomaly.

963 C In the UK, one in 80 pregnancies is ectopic. Typically, the presenting symptom is pelvic or lower abdominal pain following a recent missed period.

964 A As 75% of women with endometrial cancer are postmenopausal, the most common symptom is postmenopausal bleeding. Risk is increased by obesity, nulliparity and late menopause. Many clinicians believe that a vaginal ultrasound should be the first diagnostic procedure because it is less invasive than endometrial biopsy.

965 H More than 99% of cases of cervical cancers are thought to be caused by the human papilloma virus (HPV). In September 2008, the NHS launched a vaccination programme for HPV. The vaccine provides protection against the two types of HPV that cause cervical cancer.

966 G Endometriosis is typically seen during the reproductive years. It occurs in 5%–10% of women. It is a common cause of infertility.

The most common symptom is pelvic pain. The only way to diagnose endometriosis is by laparoscopy or other types of surgery with lesion biopsy.

967 F Cervical ectropion is indistinguishable from early cervical cancer, therefore further diagnostic studies, e.g. Pap smear +/– biopsy must be performed for a differential diagnosis. Usually no treatment is indicated for clinically asymptomatic cervical ectropions. Hormonal therapy may be indicated for symptomatic erosion.

968 B The fact that the mass is mobile excludes a bony lesion. The most likely cause in this case is a salivary gland tumour. About 85% of salivary gland tumours occur in the parotid glands, followed by the submandibular, and about 1% occur in the sublingual glands. About 75%–80% are benign. They are usually slow growing, mobile and painless.

969 F The history is suggestive of laryngeal cancer, while the neck swelling is most probably due to metastatic lymphadenopathy. Nasopharyngoscopy provides a direct view of every part of the upper respiratory tract from the nasal passages down the throat to the vocal cords. It is an invaluable part of the investigation of many conditions from hoarseness and sore throat to lumps in the neck, nose bleeds and snoring.

970 D Pain and swelling of a salivary gland is characteristic of salivary calculi. Diagnosis can be confirmed by X-ray (80% of salivary gland calculi are visible on X-ray), sialogram or ultrasound.

971 C Those features are suggestive of a carotid artery aneurysm, which can be diagnosed by digital subtraction angiography (DSA). DSA is a form of digital radiography that delineates blood vessels by subtracting a digitised tissue background image from an image of tissue injected with an intravascular contrast material with a high content of iodine that attenuates X-rays.

972 E Thyroid ultrasound may be helpful where there is a suspicion of a distinct or suspicious nodule within a multinodular goitre, to define the anatomy of the goitre prior to surgery in some cases, or where the aetiology of thyroid dysfunction is unclear, e.g. between nodular goitre and Graves' disease in a toxic patient.

973 J The cornerstone in the assessment of a solitary thyroid nodule is a procedure known as fine-needle aspiration biopsy.

974 F The classic history of anorexia and periumbilical pain followed by nausea, right lower quadrant pain and vomiting occurs in only 50% of cases of appendicitis. Pain migration from the periumbilical region to the right iliac fossa is the most discriminating feature of the patient's history.

975 C Elevated serum amylase and lipase in combination with severe abdominal pain often trigger the initial diagnosis of acute pancreatitis. Serum lipase rises 4–8 hours from the onset of symptoms and normalizes within 7–14 days after treatment. If the lipase level is about 2.5 to 3 times that of amylase, it is an indication of pancreatitis due to alcohol. Other biochemical features include hyperglycaemia and hypocalcaemia.

976 G Charcot's triad is a set of three common findings in cholangitis: abdominal pain, jaundice and fever.

977 A Pain radiating to the epigastric region is frequent with myocardial infarction, particularly with posterior or inferior myocardial infarction.

978 D Abdominal aortic aneurysms occur most commonly in individuals aged 65–75 years and are more common among men and smokers. Symptomatic and large aneurysms, i.e. those > 5.5 cm in diameter, are considered for surgical repair.

979 G This is known as the triple therapy. If the patient is allergic to penicillin, then metronidazole may be used.

980 F The standard treatment is a single dose of fluconazole (750 mg). Alternatives include itraconazole or nystatin.

981 A Piperacillin is not absorbed orally, and must therefore be given IV or IM. Other options for treatment of *Pseudomonas* infections include ticarcillin and carbenicillin.

982 C There are > 100 organisms which can cause community-acquired pneumonia. Common organisms include *Streptococcus pneumoniae*, *Mycoplasma pneumoniae*, *Chlamydophila pneumoniae* and *Haemophilus influenzae*. Healthy outpatients without risk factors may respond to a macrolide, e.g. azithromycin or clarithromycin. However, outpatients with underlying illness and/or risk factors require a combination of a β-lactam, e.g. augmentin and a macrolide.

983 J Aspergillosis is the name given to a wide variety of diseases caused by fungi of the genus *Aspergillus*. The most common forms are allergic bronchopulmonary aspergillosis, pulmonary aspergilloma and invasive aspergillosis. It develops mainly in individuals who are immunocompromised, as most humans inhale *Aspergillus* spores every day without having symptoms. Antifungals used in its management include amphotericin B or itraconazole.

984 H Metronidazole or tinidazole are effective in killing invasive amoeba. Paromomycin is the most effective agent in intestinal infections.

985 I Most females suffer from at least one episode of candidal vulvovaginitis at some point in their lives, but it is most common during pregnancy and between the ages of 20–40 years. Treatment is usually with topical clotrimazole or miconazole (either as a cream, pessary or both). In severe or recurrent infections, a single dose of fluconazole (150 mg) could be added.

986 E Acyclovir five times daily or famvir once daily may be used in management of herpes labialis (cold sore).

987 L Budd–Chiari syndrome is an uncommon condition caused by obstruction to hepatic venous drainage. It is characterised by hepatomegaly, ascites and abdominal pain. It most often occurs in patients with underlying thrombotic tendency, e.g. myeloproliferative disorders, pregnancy, malignancy, chronic inflammatory diseases, clotting disorders and infections. Management includes anticoagulation, antithrombolytic therapy, percutaneous transhepatic balloon angioplasty (PTBA) and management of ascites.

988 G Pancreatic cancer is notoriously difficult to diagnose in its early stages. At the time of diagnosis, 26% of patients have regional spread. The relative 1-year survival rate for pancreatic cancer is only 24%, and the overall 5-year survival is 5%. Eighty per cent of pancreatic cancers are adenocarcinomas of the ductal epithelium.

989 H Gilbert's syndrome is the most common hereditary cause of unconjugated hyperbilirubinaemia and is found in 5%–10% of the population.

990 B Primary biliary cirrhosis is an autoimmune disease of the liver featuring cholestasis, scarring, fibrosis and cirrhosis. It is characterised by raised antimitochondrial, antinuclear antibodies.

991 I Haemochromatosis, particularly in males, may present with the following clinical features: diabetes mellitus, liver cirrhosis, cardiomyopathy, arthritis, testicular failure, and tanning of the skin. The condition is relatively common among Celts, with a prevalence of 1% and a carrier rate of 10%.

992 D Aflatoxins are produced by many species of *Aspergillus*. Aflatoxins are toxic and among the most carcinogenic substances known.

993 A Nitrosamines are chemical compounds used in the rubber industry, cosmetics and pesticides. They are found in tobacco smoke.

994 I A study in Taiwan concluded that betel nut usage increases oral cancer risk 28-fold.

995 M Benzene is a known carcinogen and is commonly used in rubbers, pesticides and drugs. A majority of those who have been exposed to benzene have developed some form of leukaemia.

996 H Naphthylamine is an aromatic amine. It is used to make dyes. It is a known carcinogen and has largely been replaced by less toxic compounds. However, it is also found in cigarette smoke.

997 C Once a patient has become infected by herpes virus, the infection remains for life. The initial infection may be followed by latency with subsequent reactivation. Herpes viruses infect most of the human population and persons living past middle age usually have antibodies to most of the herpes viruses with the exception of human herpes virus type 8.

998 B There is a certain link between ultraviolet rays and increased risk of development of melanoma. As a result, the WHO reclassified tanning beds in 2009 as carcinogenic.

999 G There is currently an HPV vaccination programme in the UK.

1000 E At least three types of lymphoma have a definite link to EBV infection. Another cancer that can be caused by EBV infection is cancer of the nasopharynx.

Index

Page numbers to each heading are given in the following format: 'Question' locator / 'Answer' locator.